Healers on Healing

This **New Consciousness Reader** is the first in a series
of collections of original and classic writing
by renowned experts on the quest for human growth
and the transformation of the spirit.

Healers on Healing

Edited by Richard Carlson, Ph.D.,
and Benjamin Shield

Foreword by W. Brugh Joy, M.D.

JEREMY P. TARCHER, INC.
Los Angeles

Library of Congress Cataloging in Publication Data

Healers on healing.

 1. Holistic medicine. 2. Therapist and patient.
3. Love—Psychological aspects. 4. Healing—
Psychological aspects. I. Carlson, Richard, 1961-
II. Shield, Benjamin, 1952-
R733.H38   1989   613   88-24846
ISBN 0-87477-494-2

Jeremy P. Tarcher, Inc.
9110 Sunset Blvd.
Los Angeles, CA 90069

Distributed by St. Martin's Press, New York

Manufactured in the United States of America
10 9 8 7 6 5 4 3 2 1

First Edition

This book is dedicated to Dr. John Upledger, who taught me that the shortest distance between two points is an intention.

B. S.

I dedicate this book to Kristine Carlson, whose love has taught me what healing is really about.

R. C.

CONTENTS

ACKNOWLEDGMENTS

W e wish to thank each of the contributors for caring and trusting in the value of this project. We would also like to thank the following individuals for their assistance and grace in the creation of this book: Gary Doore, editor of *Shaman's Path,* for editorial assistance that turned prose into poetry; Connie Zweig, our editor at Tarcher, for believing in this project and for breaking speed and endurance records in the publishing industry; Craig Comstock, for unselfish gifts of his time and insights; David Petersen, Ray Soave, and Maria McManus, who went beyond the call of duty; and Susan Nilmeier and Kristine Carlson, who lovingly supported us throughout our obsession with this project.

FOREWORD

This book asks many of the best and most well-known nontraditional healers to distill their thoughts to the primary factor each has found to be the basis of healing. In the heartwarming sections ahead, you will have the opportunity to savor the answers to the single question they were asked: What, in your experience, is the key element or golden thread that unites healing processes? The contributors set aside secondary thoughts to present their primary realizations in an original, never-before-published manuscript.

To see this material arranged in the form of an anthology is inspiring because it offers us the perspective of many people, which no single healer, however successful, can provide. We are no longer limited to the experience of the blind men examining different parts of the elephant, unable to sense what the whole animal is like. Instead, we get a rich, multidimensional picture of healing.

As a traditionally trained physician and a creative explorer of nontraditional healing modalities, I am in a unique position to critically appreciate what is presented here. Let me put it succinctly and poetically:

Anthology literally means a gathering of flowers. I am moved and inspired by the unique beauty of each flower that makes up this arrangement, and by the profound mystery to which the arrangement as a whole brings me. I am sure you will feel the same.

W. Brugh Joy, M.D., F.A.C.P.
Feather Mountain Ranch
Prescott, Arizona

INTRODUCTION

L ife affords us occasional moments in which we may reflect upon where we are, where we have been, and where we are going. Such was the time for us one day in December 1986, in Santa Cruz, California, overlooking the Pacific.

As two Rolfers who have been trained in a variety of therapeutic techniques, we are faced daily with the limitations of our methods, as well as with their power to heal. We asked ourselves at that time what new dimension of healing might benefit the way we treat our clients.

We found many courses, seminars, and books on healing. For every new technique we learned, several more appeared at the top of our list of methods to study. We began to see that we live in a time when there are more distinct techniques, specializations, and modalities of healing than ever before.

What most therapies offer is a vehicle to deliver a very basic, potent form of healing. It occurred to us that there must be elements of healing that go beyond technique. Rather than explore the differences between these therapies, we decided to search for the common denominator, or "golden thread," that unites all healers and healing methods of ancient, current, and future times.

With this in mind, we asked healers from a variety of schools of thought to share their ideas. What we are attempting to do in this book is to help define and foster this common denominator, rather than create another vehicle to deliver it. Ninety percent of those we contacted graciously donated their time to contribute original essays.

Together they make up this extraordinary journey into healing that you are about to experience.

We believe that this anthology may be unique in its vision. Each piece is woven in to create an entire tapestry. Within this rich variety of opinion, the common strands of healing appear. You will find them as the major themes of this book: the role of love, returning to wholeness, listening to our innate wisdom, the nature of the healing relationship, the proper healing attitude, and the realization that healing is our natural state.

Each contribution is written in a "user-friendly" style that comes as much from the heart of the author as from the head. The essays will challenge you to go beyond the boundaries and limitations of particular techniques and schools of thought, leading you to explore the underlying universals on which all healing rests.

We have participated in this project as an expression of our desire to grow as therapists and to offer what we can back to the healing community. It has changed not only our work but our lives as well.

This is a nonprofit project, and profits from this anthology will be directed toward research and programs based on the nature of this book. We hope it will affect many lives in a positive way.

BENJAMIN SHIELD
RICHARD CARLSON

Part One

LOVE IS
THE HEALER

The day will come when,
after harnessing the winds, the tides, and gravitation,
we shall harness for God the energies of love.
And on that day,
for the second time in the history of the world,
man will have discovered fire.

Teilhard de Chardin

L ove is seen as one common denominator that underlies and connects all successful healing. Without it, there can be no true healing. For healing means not only a body without disease or injury, but a sense of forgiveness, belonging, and caring as well.

While the term *love* is often used loosely in the healing arts, the contributors in this section explain how and why love actually enters the process. To each contributor, healing is incomplete without genuine love, both for the person to be healed and for the healer.

Through personal anecdotes as well as scientific reports, these healers explain love as a healing tool in a way that touches us all. By incorporating the attitudes expressed in this section, we can begin to get a sense of how, with enough love for ourselves and for those to be healed, we can expand our definition of what healing is about.

Bernie Siegel

LOVE, THE HEALER

Bernie Siegel, M.D., F.A.C.S., has a private practice in general and pediatric surgery in New Haven, Connecticut. He is founder of a therapy program called Exceptional Cancer Patients and has numerous affiliations with medical and psychological associations. He is author of the best-selling book Love, Medicine, and Miracles.

As a surgeon I have worked for many years with patients suffering from life-threatening and debilitating diseases. In the course of this work, I have discovered that if such people can be brought to love themselves, some incredibly wonderful things begin to happen to them, not only psychologically but also physically. The by-product of their improved psychological attitude is a corresponding physical improvement. So, for me, the most important focus of therapy is that of teaching people how to feel and express love. And this, I have found, depends on my ability to love them and show them they are lovable.

Why is love so important in healing? Simply because it is the most significant thing in human life. Genuine love must be given freely, of a person's own free will. Love is not something that can be taken for granted; it cannot be assigned as a task. It is boring and insignificant if one is "forced" to love (which is really an impossibility). Loving has to be chosen deliberately.

This possibility of choosing to love is what makes our having free will worth the risk of its abuse—even worth taking the chance of nuclear destruction and other potential catastrophes. For when we use our freedom properly and choose to love, then love becomes tremendously meaningful because it comes from our deepest essence, the source of all freedom. Then we can feel love, and others can feel it too, so deeply that it has an actual physical effect. There is a physiology of love; it is not just an emotional experience but a whole-body experience.

For this reason I believe that love is the golden thread that unites the many forms of healing. But this is a very abstract concept, and we need to see in a more practical way how love enters into the process of therapy. Let's consider an example.

When people come into my office suffering from cancer, it is often apparent that, short of putting a gun to their heads, they are on a quick course of killing themselves—abusing tobacco, alcohol, and drugs, and working very hard at dying. In such cases I do not say, "Don't smoke," or "For God's sake, lose weight, exercise, and take your medicine." Instead I say, "I care about you and I love you. Here are some ways you can help yourself and find love for yourself. I'll see you in two weeks."

If they return without having done a thing, I still say, "I love you." I give them a hug and say again, "I'll see you in two weeks." Through that love, they begin to say, "I want to thank you for loving me. I'm beginning to love myself. I'm starting to take care of myself." They begin to ask what else they can do for themselves.

At this point I tell them about group therapy meetings and say they are welcome to attend if they don't mind talking about their lives and sharing their feelings. After this I may suggest art therapy, books to read, or certain self-image exercises—for example, sitting naked in front of a mirror for twenty minutes twice a day and saying, "You have beautiful eyes, you have a lovely smile, and I love you." Or I may mention meditation, prayer, music, and laughter.

At some point the patient suddenly realizes, "I know I'm never going to be perfect, but it's wonderful working toward it!" This is what I call growing and blooming and becoming the blossom. Patients discover that they are a seed with vast untapped potential, just waiting to sprout. Then their perspective becomes, "Wow, look what I can grow into!"

Healing through love also can be described as helping people get back on the path of their own lives. Each of us seems to be born with a "blueprint" that not only turns us into a certain type of physical being, but also maps out the path of our psychological, intellectual, and spiritual development as well. When we deviate from that inner blueprint, it often takes a psychological or physical illness to get us back on course, as if saying to us, "Hey, you're not being the best person you can be. Get back on your path."

Psychiatrist Milton Erickson tells a story about finding a horse when he was a child. Erickson jumped on the horse and rode it five miles up the road, where it wandered onto a farm. The surprised farmer asked, "How did you know how to get back here with my horse?" Erickson replied, "I didn't know, the horse knew. All I did was keep him on the road." This is how one conducts psychotherapy as well. When it is done well, the client is merely put back in touch with his or her internal blueprint and begins to follow the right path again.

Sometimes, of course, we have trouble finding the way back, and then we need help. We need someone kind enough to give us a little kick to get us moving. In therapy this takes the form of confrontation, or what I call *care-frontation,* a loving confrontation between client and therapist that in many ways is like the confrontation between horse and rider: The rider loves the horse but gives it a little kick in the side now and then to keep it moving.

If we listen to our insides, we will also find that inner therapist who says, "Pay attention! I'm going to make you hurt a bit now so you will wake up." For this reason I sometimes call pain and suffering "God's reset button." It is sometimes the only thing that will make people change.

Many external factors, of course, may contribute to our falling away from the path that is right for us—parental conditioning, peer pressure, and the like. But to get back on the path always means finding the way in which we can best contribute love to the world. For we all have our own individual way of expressing love, and when we discover what it is, then we will live the longest, be the healthiest, and enjoy life the most, as well as become able to receive the most love from others. For this reason, therapy must aim at helping clients rediscover their own unique paths of love.

Success in this work demands that the therapist find practical ways of tapping into his or her own love on a continuous basis, for without that reliable contact, the effectiveness of therapy is severely hindered. I have found three factors to be relevant to the therapist's quest for access to the inner resources of love: (1) the attempt to live one's own message; (2) the inspiration of courageous clients; (3) the awareness of one's own mortality.

Perhaps most importantly, a therapist must live his or her own message. By this I do not mean that one must be perfect. I like the way Elisabeth Kübler-Ross puts it: "I'm not okay, you're not okay, but that's okay." We are not perfect, but we can forgive each other for our imperfections. This means that in living my own message I must forgive myself for not being perfect, just as I forgive my patients. It means, too, that I will participate in the daily meditation, music, prayer, affirmations, exercise, diet, and all the other activities that our therapy groups do, because in this way it is easier for me to forgive my patients and to forgive myself.

For me, living my message also means that it is okay to work on my own wounds and to be vulnerable with the people I am caring for. In this way, my patients become my greatest resource. I can ask them to hug me if I'm having a tough day. It is not necessary to be superman. I can admit my mortality and humanness.

In this sense I am not a traditional therapist. I don't mind having body contact with patients, because they understand that this is love on a level that is safe. They know I love them in a way that has nothing to do with sexuality and is nonthreatening.

A colleague of mine, a psychiatrist, had been working for three years with a severely burned woman, trying to teach her that she was lovable in spite of her scars. After hearing me lecture on this subject, he told me, the next time the woman came in, he went over and hugged her. He said she improved more with that hug than with three years of therapy.

So there are times when body contact is appropriate. And if you really love the world, you don't have to worry about loving and hugging. If I love everybody in the hospital, I don't have to be concerned about hugging a nurse or a patient. Nobody will say, "Hey, what's he doing?" They know, "Oh, he loves everybody, so it's okay."

In my view, therapists need to learn these lessons: It's okay to love. It's okay to touch when the client is ready to let you. It's okay to let the love come back. And, if one is having a tough day, it's okay to tell the client, "I'm having a tough day today. I need a hug."

Similarly, the healer or therapist should not regard anger as something unhealthy or abnormal. Indeed, anger can be positive. If the operating room turns your world upside-down and you feel angry, it's okay to say something. People will allow you to have angry feelings, because they have them too, and they know what you are experiencing. By expressing the anger, by saying how you feel about yourself and your needs, you don't build up resentment against others. After you are done expressing yourself, you are ready to hug others and laugh with them again. Then you all know where you stand, you do not trample on each other's feelings, you respect each other, and you move on.

It is *unexpressed* anger that is harmful. Too many people confuse anger with resentment. Anger can be positive, whereas festering resentment can cause people to become murderous. It is the things we have never said that harm us most. For then our temper becomes hair-trigger and we may explode over some insignificant item with a reaction out of proportion to the cause.

Living your own message also involves an aspect of openness and humility. As a therapist, you are not seated at some remote vantage point looking down on the ignorant masses in need of help. You just do whatever is necessary, trusting that love will show what is necessary. This means not setting yourself up as an infallible expert with all the answers. Rather, it means regarding the healing process as a dialogue and a learning experience for both patient and therapist. So, if patients want to call me Bernie, it's okay. I don't have to be "Dr. Siegel." I don't have to protect myself with barriers that get in the way of helping patients open up to love.

In this way, therapy becomes a process in which client and therapist heal each other's pain. It is vital to keep in mind that you must genuinely look at your own pain and deal with it, not merely give advice without living it, without knowing how difficult it is for the client. Love will only be authentic when it comes from living experience; and if it is not authentic, it will not be convincing.

Another important facilitator of love in the therapeutic process is the fact that in this kind of work we are daily surrounded by people who are an inspiration. We see people affirming life in the midst of debilitating or life-threatening diseases, such as the courageous AIDS patient who is challenged rather than defeated by his disease, and the cancer patients who still choose to love the world, saying that their disease is a gift and their cancer a beauty mark. Such people are heartening. They keep you going and prevent you from burning out.

Yet if you get to the point where you are not loving what you are doing as a therapist, then it is better not to do it. I like to quote George Halas, the late owner and coach of the Chicago Bears football team, who lived into his eighties. One Sunday a colleague discovered him working in his office and said, "George, at your age what are you doing working on Sunday?" Halas said, "It's only work if there's someplace else I'd rather be." In the same way, if I feel there is someplace else I would rather be, I say so to my clients. I tell them that I cannot always see them.

For example, one woman had flown all the way from Georgia to Connecticut to see me. She got caught in a snowstorm and called my office on Friday afternoon to say she could not make the appointment until 7 or 8 P.M. I told her, "I can't see you then. I've got to go home. I have to fly tomorrow." She was furious, but I firmly suggested that when she got to her hotel she should call me again. When she did, we talked some more and she calmed down. I said, "Look, there are other people you can see. Maybe you're supposed to spend the weekend in New Haven." I told her I would see her on Monday evening and that I would stay until midnight then if she needed me.

As it turned out, everything that happened to her over the weekend was so positive that by Monday she regarded it as a great experience. It was better that I did not see her on Friday night, for then I would have resented her for being there. It was better that I said no. This is a difficult lesson for many therapists to learn—when to say no. We should remember that we are not going to live forever, and therefore we must say no at certain times. Then saying no is not something negative; it is actually a matter of saying yes to yourself. A healer does not always have to be at the beck and call of the world.

Lastly, love in the therapeutic relationship is facilitated by the knowledge that we are mortal, that we are all going to die someday no matter how much we jog or love or eat organically grown vegetables. With this awareness I make the most of my life in the present moment, doing today what I would most like to do with the rest of my life. My attitude is that if I should die tonight or tomorrow, my life has been complete; I have been fulfilled because I have loved fully. This is part of the message I share with people at workshops: the sense that we can use our own mortality in a positive way to get the most out of life.

Therapists also need to develop the idea that death is not a failure. In traditional medical training, of course, success is measured in terms of removing disease, or "curing," and therefore a patient's death is regarded as a failure. But with this attitude we start to distance ourselves from patients, losing sight of ways to help them in their transition through death.

It is not always possible to cure; AIDS reminds us of this. Fifty years ago diphtheria took many lives; in another fifty years no doubt we will have some new disease that resists treatment. People are always going to die, to have incurable illnesses; but they will also always have disorders that *can* be healed.

I tell people, healthy or not, that they should live as if they were going to die at any moment. Then it is easy to help others, because there is never a point at which such advice is no longer valid. You say you are going to die tomorrow? Fine, then live as if you were going to die tonight. Then, who knows, you might feel too good to die tomorrow. Or you may indeed die because you are tired and feel like going. We have much more control over the time of our death than most people realize. It is all right to die if that is what one needs to do. Because everybody dies someday, dying can't be a failure. With this attitude, death can be a healing.

Of course, there is always grief when we lose a loved one. But we must learn to take that pain and to love others with it. Consider those who have lived ninety, ninety-five, or one hundred years. They may have lost their spouses, their children, and many other loved ones. Yet after such terrible losses, people find the strength to go on, because they learn to love others. We cannot outlive everyone we love if we choose to keep loving new people. This is what survivors do: They roll the love on continuously. Thus healing, like love, becomes a never-ending process.

Hugh Prather

WHAT IS HEALING?

Hugh Prather is a crisis therapist, columnist, and minister of The Dispensable Church in Santa Fe, New Mexico. His books include Notes to Myself, I Touch the Earth/The Earth Touches Me, The Quiet Answer, *and* Notes on How to Live in the World . . . and Still Be Happy. *His latest book, coauthored with his wife, Gayle, is* A Book for Couples.

M y childhood introduction to healing was almost as conflicted and confused as the array of present-day pronouncements on this subject. On my mother's side of the family was a long line of M.D.'s, whereas on my father's side was a line of Christian Scientists. There is still within my memory bank a litany of arguments over what turns out to be a meaningless question: Which approach is right?

As a teenager I became a Christian Science practitioner, listing myself in the Yellow Pages, and was put on probation at Principia College for healing at too young an age. As a result of this and other disillusioning experiences, for a time I rejected metaphysics in favor of a strictly nutritional approach to health. Later, I began studying the metaphysician and healer Joel Goldsmith, attended born-again healing groups, and looked into a succession of hypnotic, psychic, and visualization approaches. For several years, before my wife, Gayle, and I began helping couples, Dr. Gerald Jampolsky and I gave workshops together, addressing hospital and medical groups and working with children in pain.

In short, it has taken me a half century of divergent experiences to realize that all approaches heal the body in the identical way; the only difference is in how they limit their options. So let's first consider some of the more hindering biases in this area.

The great mistaken assumption is that healing means a physical change for the better. It is believed that part of the body is healed and part is not, and that we know the difference. We have silly and arbitrary definitions of sickness because we judge sickness as undesirable and unnatural, even as an indication of inadequate spiritual effort. Consequently we want to avoid all signs of it in ourselves. Red and swollen eyes from the flu are illness. Red and swollen eyes from "a little friendly competition" are not. To have food poisoning is to be sick, but to take offense and infect one's mind with grievances is not.

In *Notes on How to Live in the World . . . and Still Be Happy* I tell about the time I was at a party in Santa Fe and a man who had arrived on a mammoth motorcycle nodded at my bandaged forehead and asked, "Dirt-bike injury?"

"No," I said, "I had a small tumor removed." I watched his features drop as fast as his opinion of me.

Why should a lesion from a dirt-bike injury indicate a more manly character than a lesion from a surgeon's scalpel? Why should the mind be somewhat proud of a leg injury from a marathon or a karate practice and somewhat embarrassed by a leg affected by bursitis or a gout attack? By general agreement one is illness and the other is not, and no one claims to heal joggers or bikers. And yet I know from my own past personal addiction that jogging can sometimes be an isolating and selfish activity, very much in need of healing, whereas the only saint I have ever known had crippling arthritis and possibly had transcended the world because of it.

When conditions fall within our notion of illness, we believe they are in need of healing. Once they are changed to fit our current picture of health, we believe the need for healing stops. A *judgment,* therefore, dictates when healing efforts begin, the target at which they are directed, and when they have accomplished their goal.

I am not making a plea for "healing the whole person," but merely pointing out that no one can say in advance which changes a person needs or which bodily conditions are best. If this point were accepted, then we would understand why the healer can heal at one time and not at another. When the body becomes the major concern of the mind, the mind cannot fulfill its potential. Healing, if it is to have any lasting effect, must serve the mind and not be a tool of judgment, comparison, and classification.

If our highest duty is to follow wholeness, peace, and the kindness of our being, to treat others fairly, and to help where we can help, then the condition of the body is only meaningful as it makes concentration on love easier or more difficult. Healing is therefore accomplished through love and *is* love. And love is the uniting principle in all healing approaches—insofar as they truly heal. Healing's opposite is judgment, and any system (or practitioner) of healing loses its effectiveness when it becomes judgmental.

The pronouncement that cancer is caused by an inability to love, or that colds are signs of lack of joy, or that AIDS is a manifestation of sinful-mindedness would not be made in the first place if we had not already judged illness as wrong. What has been accomplished in seeing that the individual plays a part in "choosing" a particular physical condition, if it is assumed that the choice is bad, weak, or spiritually inferior?

When one turns one's thoughts to what has been traditionally called God (to one's Source, to love), a shattered mind can be restored to wholeness. What greater healing could there be than this? When one turns one's thoughts to God, the soul can be purged of bitterness. What greater healing could there be than this? And many people can only turn to God when they are very sick, some only when they are dying.

It took an unsuccessful operation for terminal cancer, with an aftermath of continuous pain, for my mother to have her first deeply transforming spiritual experience. She told me that shortly after the operation she found herself in a place where others had died, a place where she could look back on the world and see how meaningless were the concerns in which people embroiled themselves. She was happy and at peace, and she somehow knew that she could either "stay" or "come back." Her choice was to return and heal the relationship with her son, whom she had abandoned as a young boy. And this she did even though she was disfigured and in increasing pain until she died two years later.

I cannot believe that it would have been better for her to have been "healed" of the cancer instead of having the operation. To have the slightest contact with her during those months was to feel the presence of God. She became another person, one who was open, happy, and utterly unselfish, one who could and did heal the hurts of a lifetime.

What constitutes the work of a lifetime, and who is to say what physical condition will help or hinder its completion? The problem with merely patching up bodies is that, as Joel Goldsmith said, "You don't know who you are putting back on the streets." The true healer merely gives the gift of healing but does not watch over the patient to say in what form it is to be received. This approach frees the healer to heal wholeheartedly, unhampered by anxiety over the possible results. Where there is anxiety, there can be no love. One of the fifty "principles of miracles" stated in Helen Schucman's *A Course in Miracles* is, "Miracles are expressions of love, but they may not have observable effects."

It was Goldsmith's observation that most healers lose this faculty within three years. (Unfortunately, many then turn to blame or artifice to maintain their image.) In my opinion, the primary cause of this loss is the healer's judgment against illness, which produces a growing egotistical pride. Illness thus becomes very real and powerful, as does any part of the world that is attacked within the mind, and eventually these healers find themselves subject to the same laws of belief as anyone else. One cannot fight something without joining with the *reality* that is presupposed in its values.

Of those healers who do not lose their ability, it is significant how many decide to give up healing later in life. Once again, this is not because they see that changing the body is bad, but because they recognize that without love it is meaningless. Often healers begin to sense that, to the public, they are merely on a list of experiments to try, like a new and somewhat suspect product on a drugstore shelf. Sometimes the simplest way to end this role is to withdraw the product (i.e., the healing) from the market.

Others, however, make healing part of an overall program of deep inner growth so that, like conscious breathing, chanting, praying, service, or any other yoga, healing becomes merely a way of opening the heart to Being, to Love. I have one friend who heals at the moment of the client's greatest and purest inner effort. This man heals with his hands. The client's eyes are closed so that the physical change (often a release from pain) is experienced inwardly and as an outgrowth of the client's determination to forgive, to commit, to bless, or to perform some other loving act. He demonstrated his approach to me (in a hotel lobby!) and I had no sense of anything being done *to* me; I felt that my own efforts (in this case to commit to the happiness of one of my sons) caused the change.

Many individuals are capable of creating an atmosphere in which the patient can change his or her unconscious beliefs, but goodness is not a necessary component at either end. Although the bodily changes we call healings are not the automatic result of bringing the mind into accord with ultimate truth, they are the result of changing the mind. For example, if one *believes* that to experience the peace of

God will change a particular physical state, then, quite naturally, this is the result. Belief, however, is not primarily conscious. Simply saying that one believes, or trying very hard to believe, or conscientiously following a prescribed course of mental imagery, verbal arguments, mystical or religious invocations, movements, silences, sounds, etc., will not necessarily change one's deeply held unconscious beliefs. Most readers of this anthology probably have experienced this for themselves.

Very few are in a position to know—with complete clarity and understanding—their own or another's unconscious beliefs. They therefore do not know perfectly what they are trying to change or even when they have changed it. All that healers can do is do the best they can. They must concentrate on healing the dark, damaged, fearful images within their *own* minds, and if the results do not look like healing, they must be certain not to fall into the all-too-common trap of blaming themselves or the patient. The instant their minds begin attacking, true healing becomes impossible, because they have betrayed their calling.

To truly heal, to deeply and permanently affect the mind, a healer must have no goal but innocence—to see it and to be it. To accomplish so great a feat, the mind has to shift away from mere pictures and beliefs to the quiet, still knowing that is love. Harmlessness, absolute and complete, is the ultimate power. When healers immerse themselves in harmlessness, what to say and what to do is gently known.

The mind that sees itself as whole and another as sick unquestionably requires healing. True healing is thus expressed within the mind of the healer and not within the body of the patient. When a healer sees that he or she is not separate from the patient—and only love holds this vision—healing is already accomplished. The mind that no longer struggles to contrast itself with another, but looks happily upon its oneness with all living things, has moved into that level of reality where healing is a constant. The healer has now received and accepted the only thing that can be given away.

One of the loveliest and most complete statements of healing I have read is a poem by Helen Schucman, the scribe of *A Course in Miracles.* I will summarize and end with it.

> To heal, it is not needful to allow
> The thought of bodies to engulf your mind
> In darkness and illusions. Healing is
> Escape from all such thoughts. You hold instead

Only a single thought, which teaches you
Your brother is united with your mind,
So bodily intrusions on his peace
Cannot arise to jeopardize the Son
Whom God created sinless as Himself.
Think never of the body. Healing is
The thought of unity. Forget all things
That seem to separate. Your brother's pain
Has but one remedy; the same as yours.
He must be whole, because he joins with you,
And you are healed, because you join with him.

Jack Schwarz

HEALING, LOVE, AND EMPOWERMENT

Jack Schwarz is an internationally known teacher, author, and research pioneer in the voluntary control of mind-body processes and enhanced states of consciousness. He is founder and president of Aletheia Foundation in Ashland, Oregon, and author of The Path of Actions, Voluntary Controls, *and* It's Not What You Eat, But What Eats You.

I believe that the common denominator of all healing methods is unconditional love—a love that respects the uniqueness of each individual client and empowers the client to take responsibility for his or her own well-being.

Whenever we fail to align ourselves with the process of transformation, we are in a stagnant state, holding back the flow of life energy, which manifests as disease. Then, by labeling our condition as disease, we often stop seeing it as an evolutionary process and come to regard it as some alien enemy attacking us from the outside. But this very attitude further constricts the flow of life energy. Hence, one aspect of the healer's love is to help the client overcome the fear of change.

Yet there can be no willingness to transcend the fear of change unless one first has the appropriate motivation to live. In my view, no one comes into this world without a function or without the tools to fulfill that function. One of the best reasons for staying healthy is to express that function to its fullest extent. So, if we are unclear about what that function is, our motivation to stay healthy will be diminished.

Thus people often need to have their attention drawn to the untapped potentials they have not yet fulfilled, either because of a particular belief system, because they have been holding back, or simply because of a lack of awareness. In any case, by drawing attention to these potentials, therapists can help people clarify their purpose and strengthen their will to live. This is one of the most powerful therapeutic tools used, in one way or another, by all successful healers, whatever their particular system or technique.

Indeed, technique is actually just a form in which the therapist's unconditional love can be transferred. We need to begin developing more faith in the process of transfer than in the particular technique used to bring it about. Certainly it has been a problem in the healing professions that we have gotten stuck in techniques. We have become such fantastic technicians that each individual is almost regarded merely as a subject for the practice of techniques. In doing so, we lose sight of the fact that each person may need a different technique, based on his or her unique needs.

But we must make it clear to people that they also have to start recognizing their own needs. This means, in my view, that therapists need to become educators. People must be given back the power to take charge of their own well-being—a power that is often taken away from them by systems of health care that tend to create dependence.

Previously, we have *over*powered people instead of *em*powering them. The real job of a therapist, however, is to give away power. By embracing clients with our own energy and excitement, we help them get their own energy stimulated, so that impediments to the free flow are dissolved in the revived surge of "current," just as we recharge a car battery that has run down. But the therapist must also educate clients in how to ignite their own engines and keep producing power so that the process continues after the healer leaves.

One disadvantage of using the word *healer* is that it can create a misconception; it implies that people should depend upon others to do their healing for them. This has been fostered by the traditional concept of the healer or therapist as an authority with privileged access to special knowledge. In the alternative model that I prefer, the healer becomes more like a mapmaker or guide, someone who "walks the territory" with clients, showing them not only the potential routes back to health, but also how to follow the trail on their own, guided by their own innate resources of healing knowledge.

In this model, the therapist does not create dependence and does not profess a monopoly of wisdom, but instead becomes a facilitator who shows people how to access their own inner wisdom and maintain certain states of energy so that transformation can take place. Thus the therapist becomes an educator in the original sense of the word, from the Latin *educare,* to "bring forth" knowledge in another person—in this case, self-knowledge.

Of course, therapists also need to develop practical skills and master specific healing and diagnostic techniques. But whatever the techniques, mastery depends on the cultivation of spontaneity, sensitivity, and intuition. For example, a skilled surgeon must be intuitive enough to recognize that if one starts cutting according to the textbook, in many cases the cut will be too close to the organs, because an individual's organs are not located exactly where the textbook shows. So, although a good surgeon may not explicitly recognize it, he or she is already intuitive, as manifested in the instinctive knowledge of when and how to cut.

There are many different ways in which we can develop sensitivity and intuition. The first and most important step is to start recognizing that everyone exists as patterns of energy and to become aware of the precise nature of the flow of energy in your own body. Beyond knowing how these energy flows work, the therapist must actually be a radiant being. Only by becoming a radiant being yourself can you know how the energy is flowing in the body of another person. The ancient injunction of Hippocrates, "Physician, heal thyself," is still a necessary foundation of the healer's art. Therapists must work on themselves if they would work effectively on others.

In my own practice, I perceive energy fields by vision and by tactile capacity. However, there are many different ways by which you can develop the capacity to sense these fields. One way is by starting to recognize the "feeling level" when you approach a person. In many cases, the physician or healer can diagnose a problem before examining the client. This comes by long practice of careful attention to the feeling level. Therapists must begin to heed and respond to the intuitive knowing that occurs at that level rather than the level of intellectualization. They must learn to recognize and trust nonverbal communication at the intuitive level.

Of course, therapists still need technical background, because they must not only be able to pick up the messages from the energy fields but also to interpret them in the appropriate way. In order to formulate a logical course of treatment, the problem must be made understandable to the rational mind, and that requires intellectual discipline. Hence there must be equal development of intellectual and intuitive faculties.

Therapists also must start to understand that one does not merely work with a physical body and its symptoms. The moment we start identifying with the body, we become dominated by it. Then the ego gets involved and we start wanting to overcome or "conquer" the problem rather than to see and understand clearly what is actually in disharmony. In the healing professions we have tended to identify the causes of disease with pathological physical states rather than with emotional and mental states. But healing goes far beyond the recovery of the body. Thus we see people treating their bodies with the most appropriate food, supplements, exercise, and so forth, yet remaining very ill.

The body is just a particular form of the universal life energy, whereas the mind is a more subtle form, which has a greater capacity for universal attunement and harmony. Thus the body needs to adapt itself to the mind. This is why the consideration of belief systems is so important in healing.

For example, we have a so-called "pathological defense system," which we call the immune system. But already this way of conceptualizing the immune system—as a *defense* system—produces an attitude that must ultimately be transcended in order for healing to occur. It is far more effective to take the attitude that we will maintain as high and exciting an energy field as possible, so that the immune system can take care of itself.

Attention to such attitudes is important because they eventually get carried over into our social life as well. For instance, if we take a defensive attitude, we tend to regard as an enemy everybody who does not agree with us. Then, as a nation we end up spending most of our national resources on armaments and preparations for war. One of the greatest aspects of healing is the realization that if we cannot be offended any longer, we have no need for defense.

As more and more people realize this, it will begin to affect the whole planet in a beneficial way, promoting the global healing we so desperately need.

Louise L. Hay

HEALER, HEAL THYSELF

Louise L. Hay, D.D., is a metaphysical counselor and teacher widely known for her workshops and books on using affirmations, visualizations, meditation, and forgiveness exercises. She is the author of the best-selling book You Can Heal Your Life.

There's a song by the Beatles that goes, "All you need is love." I believe that's true. The current of love is what flows through everything. All the healing techniques in the world won't really help unless love goes with them. So many of our problems—physical, emotional, even spiritual—come from a lack of love. I believe most people need to learn to love themselves again in order to truly heal themselves.

I find that many problems come from self-rejection and self-hatred of one degree or another. Many people, for some reason, keep creating uncomfortable experiences for themselves—through drug abuse, alcohol abuse, smoking, or food abuse, for example. Until they are willing to release the need to punish themselves, there's not a lot that can be done for them on a permanent level. Some cases may show signs of healing, but the results are often temporary.

When love is present, things are different, even with life-threatening illness. For example, it's amazing to note the changes of consciousness that have happened in the AIDS support group I work with. I see such changes all the time in everybody I've worked with.

The best thing therapists, whether medical or psychological practitioners, can do to help their clients the most is to love themselves. When therapists really love who they are, it's easy for them to teach that love to their clients. When they don't, all the talk in the world, all the methods in the world, do not really get it across.

How do we start? First, we need to stop criticizing ourselves, because criticism doesn't help—it just keeps us stuck in our problems. When we're willing to love and accept ourselves, we can make changes.

To a great extent, loving ourselves is nothing more than accepting ourselves as we are. Most of us have long mental lists of what we must do before we will love ourselves. We have to lose weight, or get a new job, or get a raise, or get a new relationship or new car or new apartment or whatever. We have all these reasons why we can't love ourselves. And if we do accomplish those things, we still don't love ourselves; we make a new list of reasons why we can't accept ourselves yet.

When we say we will love and accept ourselves as we are, it doesn't mean we're not going to change. What it means is that we're going to change by starting with the idea, "This is what I'd like to do," rather than with, "What a bad person I am to have this problem"— eating too much, drinking too much, or whatever. The positive idea, open to possibilities, is more powerful than the negative idea.

The difference may seem small, but it's important. It's the difference between feeling that we're bad or wrong, and saying "This is me as I am, and I think I'd like to change some things."

In my writings I have occasionally offered the suggestion that we consider replacing the word "should" with "could." That's really a small thing. But when people work with it, it helps to show them how rigid they often are in their thinking. Many of us have rules about how things *should be,* rather than allowing ourselves to enjoy *what is.*

We also create certain kinds of so-called illnesses within ourselves. We actually cause our minds and bodies to become out of balance to the point where they disrupt our lives. On the face of it, this is a negative thing. But there can be a benefit, a learning process that can result from illness, if we are willing to see it.

I think in many cases we can turn our problems into benefits. But I also don't think we really need to create the problems to begin with. Certainly, if we do create a problem, and then we choose to benefit from it, that's wonderful. But I think there are other ways of learning. I know it's long been a popular and even socially acceptable notion that we learn from our suffering. But, frankly, I don't think it's necessary.

I have been asked what kind of advice I might give to professionals who want to go beyond their respective techniques, whatever those might be, to find out what it is about their work that can have a deeper impact. Basically, I think that is an individual matter. But there is one aspect they could consider. I'm a simple lady and I've learned, over the years, that the one thing that makes more difference than anything else is the willingness to love ourselves. I suggest that therapists work on that as much as possible, not just look for new techniques.

I had lots of techniques myself. But it wasn't until I was willing to begin to love myself and drop the self-hatred—to live what I was teaching—that I really began getting results with people. Now, when I hold a workshop, it is really a simple workshop. If you ask the participants, "What did you do?" there's not much to tell. But if you ask them about the results that they got, that's another story.

I keep trying to show people how they are not loving themselves. Then I ask the simple question "Are you willing to let that go? Or do you want to hold on to it?" They always have the choice. And they're never "wrong" if they choose to hold on to it for a period of time.

I don't know how I began this kind of work. It just happened. When I used to work privately with clients, I was a great "fixer." I could help you fix your body, your bank accounts, your relationships, your job, and then I discovered one day that if I could teach others to love themselves, I didn't have to do all this fixing. Because if you truly love yourself, you automatically stop creating problems for yourself.

I came to the realization that somebody who really loves himself simply would not have any problems. If we do have problems in life, as all of us do, they show us where we are not yet in harmony. Helping someone discover that is the real job of a healer. It goes beyond fixing, beyond therapy.

There's no reason why this same philosophy couldn't be applied by a physician or psychotherapist. I have watched what's happened with Bernie Siegel, who wrote *Love, Medicine, and Miracles.* We worked together, so I could see it firsthand. He came out of medical school with the traditional medical mind-set. Then, over a period of time, he allowed his patients to teach him what really worked in healing. I've heard him say that the most powerful known stimulant of the immune system is love, and that love heals. We might ask, if love can stimulate the immune system, then what wears the immune system down? Perhaps someday we will find out.

I would like to see healing help create a world where it's safe for all of us to love each other. That would take care of many problems. To create this world, we each have to live it ourselves. And I think it's the therapists' obligation to do what they can to help themselves.

I never stop learning. There's always more that I can learn and more that I can release. My message is a lot like the Golden Rule: Treat others as you would like to be treated. We forget that this really means giving others the kind of love and acceptance that we ourselves would like to receive.

As children, what we wanted more than anything was to be loved and accepted as we were. That's still what all of us want, only we're not going to get it until we're willing to give it to ourselves first and then to others. To me, that's the basis of world healing. We're always pointing fingers at other groups and saying they have to do things differently. But *we* are the government, *we* are the churches, *we* are the medical profession. The changes are going to have to come through us. When enough people are willing to live that way, I think we will have peace on earth. And then we will begin to learn our real potential.

After we stop criticizing ourselves, the next step is to be gentle, kind, and patient with ourselves. We're learning many new things, and we can't learn them all in one day. I think we also need to praise ourselves a lot. Criticism breaks down the inner spirit; praise builds it up. I think we need to be loving to our negative patterns because we've created them to fulfill a need. And, if we don't put ourselves down for it, we can find a more positive way to fulfill that need.

We need to take care of our bodies, to treat them as the precious creations they are. We need to learn about nutrition and exercise. We need to look at what kind of fuel we put into our bodies and the results we get.

I'm also a great advocate of "mirror work." I think that doing affirmations and looking in the mirror and saying "I love you" is very helpful in moving us out of self-hatred. I like to ask people to get up in the morning and look in their own eyes and say, "I love you. What can I do today to make you happy?"

All these activities are simple, yet we don't practice them. When people first come to me, I ask them if they have tried even the simplest things. None of them have. I remind myself that people don't come to me because their lives are filled with joy. Then again, I am meeting more and more people who thank me because their lives *are* filled with joy now, and they feel I have been one of the stepping-stones. I really don't do anything for anybody. People do it for themselves. But they have the idea that I had something to do with helping them get what they wanted. That's what's important: that you get what you want. Who knows? Maybe it's helpful to have a stepping-stone now and then.

Serge Kahili King

REMOVING DISTRESS TO REVEAL HEALTH

Serge Kahili King, Ph.D., was trained from an early age in the Kahuna shamanic tradition of Hawaii and spent seven years studying shamanism in Africa. He is executive director of Aloha International, a nonprofit organization that is training a worldwide network of shaman healers. His best-known works are Imagineering for Health *and* Kahuna Healing.

M y philosophical background is the Hawaiian shaman system of Huna. But in my life as a healer I have explored a great many healing therapies and modalities and have noted that no matter which system is used, some people are healed with it, some are not healed with it, and some are healed without it.

What I intend to do here is express some observations made over several decades on what seems to be taking place during healing. The focus here will be on the body, but the concepts are applicable to the healing of mind, circumstance, and environment as well.

First, let's look at the fact that the body can be healed with the help of—and sometimes in spite of—an extremely varied range of methods, which I will list (only partially) in four main categories:

Physical. Herbs, drugs, and other medicines; diet and nutritional supplements; surgery and bone-setting; chiropractic and massage; deep breathing; enemas and colonics; fasting; electricity and magnetism.

Emotional. Affection and attention, laughter and play, anger release, fear confrontation, color, aroma, and music.

Mental. Placebos, hypnosis and self-hypnosis, psychotherapy, guided imagery, visualization, and affirmation.

Spiritual/Metaphysical. Pyramids, crystals, orgone devices, aura cleansing, psychic surgery, therapeutic touch, homeopathy, flower remedies, acupuncture, acupressure, applied kinesiology, telepathy, radionics, prayer, faith, positive thinking, and "spontaneous remission."

Although some of my categorizations might seem arbitrary, even this partial list is phenomenal. If the body can be healed by all these different methods—and there are countless case histories to support the healing effects of each one—then clearly each method is just a means by which the actual healing process takes place. Chemical replacement theories of the healing process are inadequate when therapeutic touch gets the same effect; surgical correction theories are inadequate when prayer gets the same effect; energy-balancing theories are inadequate when hypnotic suggestion gets the same effect; spiritual harmony theories are inadequate when nutrition gets the same effect. Therefore, let's look for a common thread in the process itself.

Before we do so, however, it is necessary to have working definitions of health, healing, and sickness. In English, *health* is defined as a condition of wholeness, or freedom from defect or separation. It is therefore akin to the word *harmony.* "To heal" means to make whole or to bring back together that which has been separated (as in healing a wound or a relationship). "To harmonize" would be a good synonym.

Cure is another word used in English meaning to eliminate a problem (such as pain, grief, trouble). Interestingly, it comes from an older word meaning "care" or "concern." Taking the basic meaning of both words into account, it would be quite proper to equate healing with loving.

Sickness (a common English word for unhealth, which is rarely used in England in that sense) basically means a state of being troubled, distressed, or grieved; *illness* means evil (which is why so many believe it is "bad" to be sick); and *disease* simply means uncomfortableness.

In Hawaiian, to which I am partial, the definitions are more clear-cut. Health is equated with energy. Good health is abundant energy *(ehuehu)*, and poor health is weakness *(pake)*, or lack of energy. Illness is equated with tension *(ma'i)*, and healing is the restoration of energy flow *(lapa'au)*. The word for harmony also can be translated as "a state of great energy" *(maika'i)*, and the word for love also can mean "to share energy" *(aloha)*.

Putting it all together for the sake of discussion, let's call health "a state of harmonious energy" and healing "to harmonize and energize." For sickness/illness/disease we'll use the word "disharmony," and for that which causes such a condition we'll use the word "distress," meaning excessive stress or tension.

At the most basic and practical level, a body is healthy to the degree that its cells are healthy. A healthy cell is one that is in harmony with its environment, has abundant energy, and is effectively performing the function appropriate to its location in time and space. To perform that function and maintain its energy and harmony, it needs a sufficient supply of nutrients and an efficient system of cleansing. If either the nutrient supply or the cleansing system is disturbed, then the cell diminishes in effectiveness, energy, and harmony and either reduces its function, performs an inappropriate function, or ceases to function at all. When the number of cells affected is enough to bring the disturbance to conscious attention by a symptom of some kind, then the body, or a portion of it at least, is declared unhealthy.

A successful healing method is one that corrects, directly or indirectly, a disturbance of cellular nourishment or cleansing. Because so many widely differing methods can do this, it will be helpful to look at the common factor producing the disturbance: distress.

Distress—constraint or tension—is what happens at the cell level when disharmony is evident. Distress, or excessive stress, constrains the flow of nutrients to the cell and inhibits the cleansing process, primarily through muscle tension. It is important to remember that some forms of muscle are used for body movement and other forms support and protect organs and nerves. So distress may not always be at a conscious level of awareness.

What brings about distress? Rather than attempt to list the physical, emotional, mental, spiritual, circumstantial, and environmental factors that may contribute to distress, let's look at the common thread here, too. Stress, whether distress or eustress (pleasurable stress), occurs as a natural effect of resistance to change. Resistance, like stress, is not bad in itself. It enables us to sense our environment, to walk across a floor, to build muscles by exercise, and to grow in many ways by working through challenges and accomplishing goals that stretch our talents and capacities for learning. But this refers to a flexible type of resistance, or a dynamic balance between resistance and nonresistance—like the kind a tree uses when it grows around a rock that it cannot break through or push aside.

Distress comes from rigid resistance, the kind that continues beyond the point of effectiveness and into the range where function breaks down. Rigid resistance takes place because of conscious or subconscious fear of whatever is being resisted. Consciously or subconsciously, a person may hold an idea that the thing being resisted is dangerous, or that the effect of not resisting it would be dangerous. Normally the body then tries to move away from the danger, to neutralize it, or block awareness of it, because the body automatically tries to reestablish harmony whenever disharmony occurs. When the existing physical or behavioral resources of the body are such that these procedures are ineffective, the continuing effort of the body to get away from or get rid of the danger results in distress. When this becomes painful enough or disharmonious enough to reach conscious awareness, the person usually seeks other methods that will hopefully be more effective.

Basically there are only two things to do about distress: either remove what is being resisted, or cease resisting it (change the reaction). All healing methods, even the spontaneous ones of the body, use one of these two methods. Surgery, for instance, may use the first method by removing an object, such as a bullet, which is being resisted by the body; or the second method by stitching separated parts of the body back together or implanting a new part. Therapeutic touch may use the first method by inducing the decrease or disappearance of a tumor, or the second method by increasing the strength or relaxation of the body. An ordinary individual uses the first method when he or she puts out a fire to avoid getting burned, while a nonordinary individual might use the second method and alter his or her body so that the fire doesn't produce a burn.

From my observation and personal experience, I am convinced that health is a natural state of harmonious energy that gets covered up or inhibited (disharmonized) by distress. Remove the excessive stress by action or reaction and health appears, because it was there all the time just waiting to manifest. Regardless of method, healing will not take place unless the energy flow of the body or cell has been restored. Removing or changing resistance will improve the flow of energy and produce or assist healing.

Many modern healing systems are often ineffective because they attempt to be overly exclusive. In other words, they tend to treat illness as being caused *only* by physical, emotional, mental, or spiritual conditions and to reject other conditions as having no bearing on the case. Yet stress can come from any of these realms and is usually mixed in particular symptoms. Even something as simple as a smashed finger can be related to feelings of guilt, or to confusion about a life direction, or to spiritual alienation, or to all of these. If the finger is only treated at the physical level, then the healing will be slowed by the distress being maintained by one of the other conditions.

A healer ignores any one of the conditions at the peril of the person who is to be healed. It frequently happens that dramatic improvement in mental health occurs through nutrition, that tumors are removed with hypnosis, and that emotional release cures spiritual apathy. Seldom can one healer be all things to one person, but love draws the right healer to the right client at the right time.

Healing can only occur because there is some harmonious state known to the body (or to the spirit of the body) that it loves so much that it will spontaneously move toward it whenever possible. Distress —caused by resistance, which is caused by fear, which is the absence of love—in its turn causes disharmony, or disrupted energy and relationships. Healing, an act of caring and loving, removes the distress and allows the body to return to the harmonious energy state it loves.

The common thread in all healing cannot be other than love, pure and simple: the love of the healer (recognized or not) for the one being healed, and the love of the healed (recognized or not) for the state of harmony and full energy. Love may be used as a method of healing, but it is always the process.

Part Two

RETURNING TO WHOLENESS

Something we were withholding made us weak
Until we found it was ourselves.

Robert Frost

W holeness or health is our natural state. The nature of healing involves removing the obstructions to this natural state and bringing individuals into alignment with themselves and their world. Free of these obstructions, an individual's innate intelligence and self-regulating capabilities will guide him toward a state of well-being.

While each of the authors takes a different approach in philosophy, in this section they see the role of the healer as guiding those who have fallen out of balance to reestablish harmony and wholeness in their lives. The authors discuss how healing can go beyond the individual's mind, body, and spirit to heal family relations and eventually even global imbalances.

Richard Moss

THE MYSTERY
OF WHOLENESS

Richard Moss, M.D., is the founder and spiritual director of Three Mountain Foundation in Lone Pine, California, a nonprofit organization for health and wholeness. He leads workshops and conferences throughout North America. He is the author of The I That Is We: Awakening to Higher Energies through Unconditional Love *and* How Shall I Live?

N one of us is indifferent to healing. When we are healthy, we rarely have a sense of the incredible dynamism of aliveness within us, nor do we appreciate that our sense of being is a fragile thing indeed. When the veil of immortality is rent by sickness, or the ego-self dissolved in a great wash of Existence, we are shocked as we could never imagine. Even rinsing the dishes can seem like a miracle.

When we have health once again, when we find ourselves poised in a renewed sense of identity, restored to capacities that make our lives meaningful, we are grateful—more than grateful. We touch ourselves as if for the first time.

Now we speak of healing. We want to understand it, perhaps share this gift with others. But what is healing? Is it merely the return to a familiar and satisfying life? I think not. To me it is the place of, as T. S. Eliot wrote, "the intersection of the timeless with time." This rapprochement is more than poetic awareness. It is an alchemy within our cells. Healing is a glimpse into the universal process of incarnation. Our very flesh vibrates with a larger connectedness to life.

When I was a traditional physician, I was content to regard

healing as the restoration of health. But today I know that healing is far more than a return to a former condition. True healing means drawing the circle of our being larger and becoming more inclusive, more capable of loving. In this sense, healing is not for the sick alone, but for all humankind.

Why is healing often coupled with suffering? This is the great drama of matter ascending toward spirit, and spirit incarnating in matter. Is our suffering the process whereby ancient memories embedded in our flesh are gradually brought to consciousness? Perhaps if there were no suffering, our bodies could be left behind in the transformational journey (as many would like us to believe). We might fly off as some ethereal spirit, and all would be blissful and perfect.

But it is far more wondrous that we do not fly off. Our consciousness grows precisely because it cannot slough off the flesh. Consciousness is called to earth as humankind, mortal. All the great metaphysical truths become alive in the transforming paradox of living. There is an enormous challenge here that we seldom face. Yet every once in a while, one of us steps authentically into the midst of this great and mysterious drama and, at such moments, there is healing. And the greatest healing brings us more fully into life.

After years of exploring the transformational process and witnessing many healings, I have drawn some insights that point toward the underlying forces of all healing modalities. Yet I should caution that any understanding can be as much a burden as a gift. In giving words to what was formerly mysterious, a certain innocence or grace is lost. No sooner is it grasped than it dissolves. In the end, healing must be a ceaseless process of relationship and rediscovery, moment by moment. The more we "know" about healing, the more we are simultaneously carried toward something unknowable. For this reason all healing is in essence spiritual.

Healing in the deepest sense is a mystery. Even modern medicine with its pretext of being scientific rests upon observations that, at their heart, are unexplained. One of the definitive texts of pharmacology begins by reminding the reader that ultimately no one knows how any drug works. Of course, the average physician conveniently chooses to forget this and actually comes to believe that he knows what he is doing.

There is no question that many of these formulations "work" predictably. Yet when we expect a certain response from a particular treatment, we are more in the business of shuffling symptoms than in the business of healing. Where mystery is denied, one can feel the growing sense of a haunting dis-ease among the medical community.

Not only do the patients fare poorly, but the physicians as well. We must ask questions and seek to understand ourselves and our world, but we must not forget that at the perimeter of our experience, at the frontier of our science and thought, there remains a vast impenetrable mystery. It is from here that I believe healing flows.

Wherever we see the emergence of a new quality of wholeness, we simultaneously witness healing. And we find unique individuals who have gone beyond the boundaries that define conventional reality. To me this is the heritage of the healer, the mystic, the shaman, the true scientist. It is really the fruits of these lives that have been "healing" humanity all along. These fruits are the root of what we call culture. Yet it is the tree of life that each of us must bring to full form in ourselves. Culture begins to die, as do we, when we unconsciously eat of the fruit of other trees. All that has been, no matter how sacred, how "proven," is but the stage from which to leap toward even greater possibility. Yesterday's healing revelation can become today's prison unless we discover for ourselves the relationship to life that forever gives birth to new fruits.

Here then, for me, is the golden thread: relationships. It is our capacity to merge, to become at one, however briefly, with ourselves, with each other, and with life in a larger sense. Healing, wherever and however it occurs, brings each person and humanity as a whole toward a more inclusive, more unobstructed relatedness to all that is emerging in this adventure of life. The relatedness is endless: to oneself, to one's sensations, thoughts, feelings, images, dreams; to other people in how we acknowledge and transcend the sense of separation. And it is relatedness to something more, however we conceptualize it: Self or God.

If we look carefully at this quality of relatedness, there seem to be three vectors that pierce through our conditioning and allow a state of harmony to arise between our instinctual and spiritual awareness. Far beyond techniques for healing or transformation, these vectors are functions of consciousness itself. As such, they transcend time or historical context. Whether you are an aborigine, a Native American medicine man, a modern physician or psychotherapist, whether you regard yourself as a healer or just an "ordinary" person, the process of healing involves the dance of these forces. I call them:

1. Creative Involvement: an original and spontaneous participation in life without judgment.

2. Intensity: the quality of attention, the depth from which our involvement with life emanates.

3. Unconditional Love: the principle of inclusivity, an implicit sense of prior wholeness.

These transformational vectors offer us new insights into the process of healing. Take, for instance, the breakthrough of Sigmund Freud. He observed the unconscious mind expressing itself in dreams and other spontaneous imagery. By helping his patients bring unconscious content into conscious awareness, Freud helped to heal certain maladies. But the heart of his achievement does not rest in his ideas and insights alone. It rests in the quality of relatedness he brought to his own psyche and to his patients.

To me, Freud's originality was that he *listened* in a new way. Not long ago I visited his home in London and stood quietly in the room where he worked with his patients. Freud would sit at the head of the couch facing away from the patient. I believe he did this so that he was not distracted by the usual visual habits that prevent real seeing. He was a collector of ancient artifacts. His room was filled with mythic statuary and symbols. There in the midst of this multicultural sense of the human adventure, he "heard" other dimensions. This way of listening in itself represents Creative Involvement.

Furthermore, he was not listening casually; he was fully attentive yet relaxed, listening from his depths—exhibiting Intensity. It might have been days or months before he made notes, because writing could prematurely lock his attention into old assumptions and old modes of understanding. In fact, his therapeutic relationships unfolded and evolved. There was room for something unexpected to happen, a quality of relationship in which consciousness could speak in new ways. It is this openness, this unspoken faith in an unrealized possibility, that bespeaks Unconditional Love.

Unlike the majority of his fellow physicians, Freud listened to the unheard and the unspoken. It is this kind of attention that every good therapist, priest, or healer brings to another, or that the original thinker brings to the conceptual structures of his time, or that the scientist brings to the phenomena he is studying. In this state of communion, a healing energy is engendered. The scriptural injunction "Where two or three or more are gathered . . . there shall I be in their midst" speaks to this phenomenon.

This quality of attention is our greatest gift to ourselves and to each other. Gathered in this way, a higher order of consciousness arises, a higher order of Self. For those who have learned to sense this energy, it is literally a felt presence. In this presence we are subtly or profoundly transformed. It is a higher energy state, and with it comes an enlargement of consciousness with a corresponding heightening of intuition and intelligence. It is as though various functions of consciousness such as feeling, thought, action, and sensation unite in a new order of psychophysical being.

We can see these principles operating everywhere. When we open *A Course in Miracles,* the Bible, a book of inspirational poetry, a scientific journal, or any source that catalyzes a shift of perspective, our relationship to our own experience shifts. In this new Creative Involvement our energy is freed. When Norman Cousins used laughter and vitamin C to heal himself, this was Creative Involvement. His commitment and wholeheartedness to his regimen represented Intensity. The very fact that he felt permission to honor his own intuitive healing sense and do what had not been done before is evidence of the underlying vector of Unconditional Love.

But a word of caution: Yes, laughter is healing. But is it as healing when someone tells us to do it as when we find laughter spontaneously emerging from within us? Similarly, new cancer treatments often have better results in the institutions in which the treatment originated than when they are repeated elsewhere. The spontaneous creative quality of a new treatment applied by the originators may carry a greater healing capacity.

To our outer consciousness, it is what is done—whether taking a medication, prayer, healer's touch, exercise, or diet—that seems to be the cause of the healing response, not the consciousness in which the action was undertaken. Even traditional medicine began with a creative new relationship to our human condition and owes its success to the universality of the scientific approach. But scientific creativity can easily become dogmatic.

In physics, when we study the particle aspect of light, the wave function collapses; a similar phenomenon happens in our search to understand healing. If we name the healing phenomenon so that we can grasp it consciously and employ it for our own ends, what we hold no longer is connected to its more universal quality. In medicine, when we have a new healing insight, we automatically begin to think in terms of application, techniques, and formulas. Thus we are on the way to freezing the universal healing force we set out to liberate.

I have spent years orchestrating high-energy human interactions and observing the resulting unification and heightening of consciousness. There are expansive feelings of love and well-being, states of mystical opening, and physical healings. First comes the deeper relationship to life in this moment, and all the rest follows.

But conscious understanding of the forces that lead to such a moment does not necessarily allow the creation of such unification on our terms, especially because healing is desired. There is an element of grace, a surrendering into life on its terms. In naming these vectors, I have tried to reach beyond the outer phenomena toward a more universal dimension. It is precisely because we cannot orchestrate these vectors on our terms that healing, or any fundamental transformation, will always remain mysterious.

I am reminded of Jesus' remark that "No man comes unto the Kingdom through his own efforts . . . and everything is possible in God." In one stroke we are offered hope and hopelessness. But I do not think we have grasped the significance of this remark. We live in a time when intellect has wrested so many secrets from every corner of existence. Similarly, we seek to do the same with our psyches, thus the endless stream of "how to's" that glisten briefly on the best-seller list, only to be replaced by the next self-improvement formula. Such efforts can involve a creative relationship to life or a compulsive manipulation of ourselves and our environment. It depends on whether we have made the discovery for ourselves and whether we are seeking to run from life to some illusion of security, or yielding ourselves into life's wonder. In either case, there comes a point when no effort consciously undertaken assures us of true healing. Our many triumphs must stand side by side with this deeper mystery in which we are humbled, even wounded in our pride.

True healing (not merely the temporary alleviation of symptoms or the apparent conquest of a disease by science) is never fully on our terms. Any original and wholehearted response to life carries the capacity to shift the energy of consciousness, and the result is transformation of one degree or another. Yet within such a spontaneous aliveness there is something that always remains unpredictable, something of faith and grace. When we apply a formula, we get a result, but often the response is transient, a shifting of symptoms, a deferment of the problem for a period of time. This is what I refer to as perturbation. For a while, there is new insight, new feeling and understanding, maybe even remission of disease. Certain diseases seem "cured." But in a deeper sense this is not healing; the circle hasn't really grown larger. We can end up even more vulnerable to a new disease, because the very process of trying to change things on our terms blinds us to listening more directly to life. We are compelled to fix, rather than to come unto the Kingdom through the agency of Life.

Wholeness is something to which we may aspire; certainly I do. I listen to my dreams, fantasies, and visions, to the signals from my body, to the quality of how I meet people in my world. I offer myself to grow in the capacity to love. I listen so I may decipher the mystery of myself and become more whole.

Yet I know that I don't know, that my own transformational moments and those that I have observed in others are not something that I can will or make happen. Like a man climbing a mountain, the vista expands far faster than our capacity to grasp it. Every new understanding elevates us so that we perceive a greater horizon. Yet it would also be correct to say that those who have had the greatest vision are in a relative sense the most ignorant. Whatever may be revealed by looking through the lens of the three vectors, healing remains a mystery and, as such, calls us forever to the new horizon of ourselves.

Lynn Andrews

MIRRORING
THE LIFE FORCE

Lynn Andrews is the author of Medicine Woman, Flight of the
Seventh Moon, Jaguar Woman, Star Woman, *and* Crystal
Woman, *which recount her training in the path of a Native American
medicine woman. She currently lives in Los Angeles, where she devotes
herself to writing, counseling, teaching, and living the Medicine Way.*

M any people today feel a strong need or desire to live in a more
whole way, to live a fuller life. That's why they seek therapy.
The question is, what do they get from therapy?

When I first met my native teacher, Agnes Whistling Elk, I had
done a lot of study in psychology. Many of my friends were psychiatrists. I had seen people go through one or another of the leading
therapies, sometimes an extraordinary process. Often they would
come out knowing why they were doing or not doing something, yet
continue in their old patterns. I asked a friend, a well-known therapist,
why he thought this occurred. He said, "We can help people to
understand why they do the things they do, but we can't necessarily
change people."

That statement was a real eye-opener for me. I thought, if therapy doesn't change you, then what is the point of it? To understand
it intellectually is just one part of the process. I had to find a way to
go on from there.

Shortly after that, I met Agnes and went to work as her apprentice. Three to six weeks later, I realized that I had manifested real change in my behavior. The ways in which I had been sabotaging myself had suddenly come to an end. I asked Agnes, "How is it that I am capable of manifesting such change in my life through working with you?"

"Partly," she said, "because the work is experiential. So often, in your society, much of the knowledge that is given to people is borrowed knowledge. You sit in a lecture hall and people tell you all these wonderful things and you take notes. The problem is that it's so difficult to make what they have told you a part of your own dream. There's no transfer of wisdom. Experience is really the link. If you could somehow experience what that person was telling you, then it would become real to you, instead of just being part of an intellectual process.

"There is one other thing," she went on, "that is really the most important. There is an added aspect of the sacred. You're not doing this shamanistic process just to clear out your head. You're doing it because you understand that to be on this earth at this time means you have chosen to evolve and to attempt to become enlightened."

The difference between shamanistic psychology and the more traditional therapies is that the first includes an aspect of the sacred. Most therapies do not talk about the process of enlightenment because their practitioners think it smacks too much of religion. Oddly enough, most of the world's religions don't talk about it, either.

The process of shamanism is the process of becoming a total being, so that you can become a teacher by example, so that in turn you can evolve into a much higher state of awareness. It's difficult to put all this into words, partly because English is a poor language to describe the process of spiritual progress. It's a pragmatic language, one that does not readily avail itself to the world of spirituality.

When you remember that a culture grows out of the language that it speaks, rather than the other way around, it's understandable why so many people in the West tend to go to the East to find knowledge. Perhaps that's also why surgery and drugs have been more important in Western medicine than the ancient knowledge of healing.

A healer does not really heal; a healer can only present a mirror. You can never really help anyone; you can only help people to see themselves. When people come to you for help, often what they are doing is looking for a way to support the neuroses they already have.

What I essentially do is to look at them as they are and give them an image of that. If the image is true, and they can see it, they can learn from it and decide if they want to change. Then I mirror an image of what they could become. What they do is their choice.

Imagine that all of us are icebergs floating on the sea of enlightenment. As an iceberg, you look down into the sea of enlightenment and know that you want to be a part of it. Then you discover that you too are made of water, except that you are frozen. You're just like the sea. The only difference is the temperature. Then, if you have the courage, you begin to wonder why you are so cold. If you become deeply involved with that question, sooner or later you will go to a teacher and ask certain questions. And the teacher will hold up a mirror. If you have the courage, you will look in that mirror and see the myriad ways in which you are losing precious life force. You are like a sieve, with many different holes through which you are losing your natural energy or heat, and so you are cold. When you close up those holes, you hold your power. You heat up, and the iceberg melts into the sea of enlightenment.

The life force pours out of you through the holes you create in your life through what I call addiction. Addictions are ways we have of fooling ourselves. In fact, the more intelligent we are, the more we can trick ourselves. If we don't smoke, drink alcohol, or take drugs, we think we're just fine because we don't have any addictions. But we may have other addictions that may be even more insidious. Usually the worst are emotional addictions, such as addiction to sadness, to chaos, to a feeling that we're not good enough.

Whatever their nature, addictions cause you to lose life force. So you decide to do something about it. You come to someone like me. My job is to show you your addictions. Then you can choose to do something about them.

I believe that all beings on this planet want to become enlightened, one way or another. Yet at the same time it's the thing they're most afraid of, usually unconsciously.

Let's say you are a smoker. People say that if you smoke, you should quit. Nobody ever asks why you have that addiction; they only deal with the fact that you have it. The reason you have the addiction is to bleed off the life force, so that there is no danger of ever becoming enlightened.

When you bleed off the life force, you are literally bleeding off heat; therefore, you get cold. When you quit smoking, for instance, and the life force you were losing is suddenly retained, you begin to get warm. It's a very unfamiliar feeling. We call it "holding your power." When that happens, when that unfamiliar feeling comes, people panic, and they look around frantically for a new addiction. A person who quits smoking usually starts to overeat or starts some other new addiction right away. They need the addiction because they've built up heat and they have to get rid of it.

When I am working with people, I can see certain things, lights or other signs of their energy field, that indicate what they're doing to themselves. I cannot just present that insight to the person—it doesn't do any good. People have to discover those things for themselves. Anyone with even a rudimentary knowledge of the mind knows that. Shamanism has a lot of psychology built into it.

Shamanism is an ancient way of healing; it has been in existence for probably a hundred thousand years. It is effective and pragmatic. In the beginning, it heals with the psychology of the individual, moving into the spiritual side later on.

I find it odd that a lot of the people who get involved with spiritual work and healing want to throw away their bodies, to reject or escape the physical plane. They think money is bad and everything that has to do with the physical plane is bad. Yet, we have chosen to be born into a physical level for a reason. We have to live consciously in the physical world. That does not mean throwing away our bodies. It means understanding our bodies and treating them with great reverence. It means learning to deal with money and other attributes of the physical life with sacredness.

There are many people practicing various therapies or techniques today. A growing number seem to be aware of the need to go beyond technique to look at what really matters, what can make their approach to healing have a real impact. I think it's very important that they introduce an aspect of the sacred into their work in some way.

Everybody sees the sacred in a different way. For some it's Judaism; for others, Christianity; still others explore shamanism. I believe shamanism is wonderful because it takes people back to the earth and to the female aspect of themselves. When we look out, we see a world terribly out of harmony. We have been living in a patriarchy, and that linear mode has put us desperately out of balance. When we talk about bringing balance back onto the earth, we are talking about the missing element, which is *feminine consciousness.* When I say that, I am not saying that woman is better than man. I am referring to *a part of our inner selves.* I simply think it's part of what we're here to do, which is bringing balance back to the earth. That is perhaps the greatest aim of healing.

When we talk about healing, we're talking about totality. There is no totality without some aspect of sacredness. As Agnes said, we come into this "earth walk" like a piece of shattered mirror, each piece reflecting the light of the Great Spirit. We spend our entire lives trying to fit those pieces back together into a cohesive whole, a working mandala.

The experiential component is crucial. Healing is not a passive process. When people come to see me for only an hour, it is difficult to generate a sense of experience in that short a time, but it is possible. Helping people discover things about themselves for themselves can be a very intensive experience.

Therapy has been enhanced significantly these past few years. More people are beginning to realize that new things have to be learned. Some therapists, of course, have trouble with the idea of introducing something called "sacred" into their work. I don't know if it's because they're atheistic or simply afraid. Either way, they make their work more difficult than it need be. On the other hand, I don't think of myself as a therapist. I do a kind of spiritual counseling. When I can, I teach. I try to incorporate everything I need into my work. As I heal, I seem to tap more into that common denominator that allows me to help other people. In other words, I become more of a mirror to other people, and it becomes easier for me to be a healing force in their lives.

The question arises sometimes about healing on a world scale. I think that world healing begins with the individual. I don't think you can go out into the world and heal, on an effective level, if you don't start at home first, with yourself, with the people around you.

I have found that it is much more important to work with one or two apprentices to see that they raise their consciousness to a high level, rather than trying to raise the level of a whole nation by being a political person. I was once very involved in Indian politics, and I found that it was not effective. It was much more effective to write books in the hope of reaching more people who can then go out and heal the people around them.

The times, too, are changing. I think that people are opening like they have never opened in their lives. As I travel, I see a great hunger and openness. People are being forced to grow. I think it may have to do with the nuclear holocaust on the horizon and with the pollution of the environment. People are beginning to realize that they have to wake up and see that the way they have been living is not adequate.

I think they're not only looking for new answers, they're also looking for new questions.

The direction of healing is going back to the earth. We are beginning to remember and understand that living in harmony with mother earth is more important than almost anything else. And, in the process of learning how to live in harmony on the earth, people will understand more about their own psyches.

O. Carl Simonton

THE HARMONY
OF HEALTH

O. Carl Simonton, M.D., is a pioneer in the use of visualization and guided imagery in the treatment of cancer. He currently practices psychosocial medicine at the Simonton Cancer Center in Pacific Palisades, California, and is coauthor of Getting Well Again *and* Stress, Psychological Factors and Cancer.

Health is the natural state of humanity. It means being in harmony with ourselves and our universe. When we are in harmony, we feel better, feel more joy, and feel healthier. If we don't recognize that state, we need to. That is what healing is all about. The more we are able to align ourselves with who we are, the healthier we are. As we work on this alignment, it prepares us for healing. I see healing as a positive feedback system and illness as a form of negative feedback.

We live in a time when there are more techniques for healing than ever before. The question we must ask is this: What is it, beyond or beneath those techniques, that really fosters the healing process?

The common denominator of healthful techniques rests on several basic questions. Does the technique bring us more in line with who we really are? Does it help us to become more in harmony with ourselves and our universe? If so, then that technique fosters healing. The degree to which it brings about harmony determines the quality of the healing and the speed at which it takes place.

It is clear that any given technique may work more effectively for one person than for another. The question of which one(s) to use is a matter of understanding who that person is and what he or she needs most. I use techniques such as guided imagery and visualization in my work. In doing so, I try to work with the person's inner wisdom, to tap the "inner physician."

Music is a good metaphor. If I were teaching music, my main objective would be to see the potential in the individual, to help bring out the qualities that are there and the traits that are easiest to access. The same is true in healing. I try to help people bring out those traits that are near the surface. This gives them energy to work on those that are more difficult to reach. I begin by looking at what is right with the person, rather than what is wrong.

We need to move in the direction of health, in the direction of who we are. I take the position that everything in the universe is trying to help us regain health and move in that direction. This is a very difficult concept for most of us to accept. When we begin to tap inner wisdom, we focus consciously on the help that is available to us everywhere we look. It is a matter of tuning ourselves and being able to hear the messages. We have to remind ourselves, however, that we cannot simply take the process for granted. It is easy to say, and yet incredibly difficult to do.

It can be done if we are open to it. The decision to be open is probably the most important single step toward healing. The concept of contacting the inner guide is one aspect of that decision. It means going inward, quieting ourselves, opening to help and asking for that help. This fosters the belief that help is available and strengthens the concept of trust.

One of the most effective ways to build belief is by using our imagination. We can imagine this communication with an inner resource and appreciate that this resource is both inner and outer. The more we imagine, the more we create a climate for a whole new view; the more we accept this new view, the more we allow understanding to begin as we practice it. That is what permits us to overcome illness.

Illness is a negative feedback system: It is telling us what we need to stop doing. If we look at illness that way, then it has great value. It might be telling us that we need to modify our work habits, to rest, or to question what we are doing. It helps us stop doing things that are counterproductive. It helps us align ourselves. It forces us to reach out for help, bringing more love to us. Illness can help us connect in a deeper, more loving, more cooperative way with people around us, rather than isolate ourselves.

Feelings about an illness are easier to change than the physical conditions. So it makes sense to me as a healer that a clue can be found in those things that improve the feelings. If we can find what makes us feel better, then the physical changes will start to occur.

The healing process is a creative process; you must be sensitive and able to improvise and draw on your knowledge as the situation unfolds. If you are tuned in, you can do whatever presents itself at the time. You can learn to follow the inner self, the inner physician that tells you where to go. Healing is simply attempting to do more of those things that bring joy and fewer of those things that bring pain. Someone once said, "Let joy be your compass heading." This means that you should follow those things that bring joy into your life. Not just superficial joy, but deep fulfillment.

Implementing this at a pace that is comfortable is very important. People often want to do things in a hurry. I'm one of those people. I recognize it quickly in my patients, because we most readily see in others those problems that exist in ourselves. I am very sensitive to the side of my patients that wants to do things too fast and to excess, because that tendency is part of my own personality.

That brings us to the question of wisdom, and in particular the wisdom of how to integrate joy and not overdo it. One of my problems is that I tend to do things I like to excess. I sail to excess; I exercise to excess; I work to excess. So I have to learn to balance. Fortunately, I have people around me to remind me when I stray and to support my efforts to regain balance. My greatest help, however, is my own awareness.

Support systems are critical. In my case, my family is a significant part of my support system. When they are not supportive, it takes a huge toll on me. When they are supportive, it enhances my life. I've been involved in a fair amount of controversy in my work. In the first three or four years of this work, my family was suspect of what I was doing and of my motivations. That was a troubling time for me. But, as my parents and siblings began to understand what I was doing and became excited and supportive of my work, they were a great resource for me. Later on, when I went through other times of controversy and difficulty, I had the family support to draw upon.

I believe that the attitudes and beliefs of the people we live with have a huge impact on what we do. For instance, in the case of illness, if my family believes that I'm going to die and there is nothing that I can do about it, this makes the process of getting well incredibly difficult. On the other hand, if they believe that I can become healthy again, their beliefs strengthen my ability to achieve it. This is true in any significant relationship, including the one between patient and healer.

The attitude of the healer is almost as important as the attitude of the person being healed. I think that's why it is important to separate the healer from the physician. You do not need any credentials to be a healer, whereas you do need credentials to be a physician. But physicians are not necessarily healers.

It is important to understand the position of the physician. This is particularly true if the physician is not a healer and does not understand the importance of attitude in healing. The physician is trained in the prevailing beliefs of the medical profession. If the patient can learn to view those beliefs as simply one person's beliefs, rather than being overwhelmed by the doctor's authority and taking those beliefs as truth, he can be more aware of the type of care he is receiving. This becomes very important in helping a person deal with a physician who believes that there is no chance for cure or even any significant chance for improvement.

If you, as a healer, can help the patient understand this, you will be doing a real service. Because you are not limited by the physician's or the health-care team's beliefs, you can help the patient get much more out of whatever treatment is being offered than the physician would even guess is possible.

We have to remember that it may be inappropriate to expect physicians to be healers when they are not trained to be. Personally, I believe that a high percentage of physicians are natural healers. Healing may, indeed, be what motivates many of us to become doctors in the first place. But all too often that gift gets trained out of us.

It does not make any difference that you are a natural healer if you aren't using any of those abilities. If you involve yourself in a profession that depends on illness for its practitioners to make a living, it is very easy to get caught up in an unhealthy role. We've heard psychologists say that they often have a vested financial interest in having their patients remain mentally disturbed in some way.

I appreciate the old Chinese system in which a physician is fired when someone gets sick. Then the physician has a vested interest in keeping you healthy. Therefore, when the doctor sees you doing something that is likely to bring on illness, it is in his best interest as well as yours to confront those behaviors and actions.

Unfortunately, that approach is just the opposite of what we have in our society today. Our physicians are rewarded when people get sick.

What direction do I wish to see healing take in the future? I would hope that it will become clearer to everyone that the purpose of healing is to bring us in harmony with our earth, with our environment, and with ourselves. As that becomes the focus, I think it will spread and have an impact on the way we view the whole idea of healing.

I want to reiterate my belief that health is a natural state of being in harmony with ourselves and our world. To achieve that, help is there, all around us. If, because of our conditioning, we can't see it, we need to relax and allow it to be revealed. To me, that is the essence of healing and the essence of who we are. It is simply opening to who we are, trusting in this process that created us, that is guiding us along.

The more I can love everything—the trees, the land, the water, my fellow men, women, and children, and myself—the more health I am going to experience and the more of my real self I am going to be.

George Goodheart

INNATE INTELLIGENCE IS THE HEALER

George Goodheart, D.C., is an adjunct lecturer at the University of Pittsburgh School of Dental Medicine and founder of applied kinesiology. He recently published the popular book You'll Be Better.

The human body has a remarkable built-in healing mechanism; it is constructed and programmed in such a way that it can heal itself. In chiropractic we speak of an innate intelligence or physiological homeostasis that automatically strives to restore equilibrium in the body when an imbalance occurs in any of its many complex systems. This innate intelligence is the common basis for all healing. People are healed by many different kinds of healers and systems because the real healer is within. The various healing modalities are merely different ways of activating that inner healer.

There is a growing body of empirical evidence that supports the idea of an inner self-correcting mechanism in the body. For instance, many scientists claim that the body is a hologram and the brain contains a three-dimensional blueprint for the structure of the body as a whole, complete to the last detail of anatomy. My own observations from working with patients support this idea. I would add, however, that besides an innate blueprint for structure, we also seem to have blueprints for both chemical and psychological normality. The body recognizes and tries to correct aberrations from these as well.

Healing occurs based on this template of healing. The body constantly compares itself to its "hardwired" programs for ideal form and function. If it notices any discrepancy between the actual and the ideal, it automatically triggers a self-correcting mechanism. The action of this mechanism then manifests as a "symptom" of some kind. Thus the process of illness is a result of the body's attempts to heal itself. This is why, especially in the musculoskeletal system, we sometimes become aware of aches and pains that confront us for a day or so and then go away. They arise because the body, having recognized an aberration, tries to fix it.

I often see this professionally as a chiropractor. One of the basic principles of chiropractic is "structure determines function." For example, many times the hipbone will have moved slightly out of alignment. The amount of movement is measured in fractions of a millimeter, yet it's like a speck of dust in the eye: The amount of irritation is out of proportion to the size of the object causing the disturbance. In such cases, examination often reveals that one limb apparently looks shorter than the other. What is really happening, however, is that the muscles are straining in an effort to put the hip back into place.

This means that the way to diagnose a problem is to carefully observe how the body is trying to repair itself. Therapy, then, consists of gently helping the body do what it is trying to do.

Another example of the body's self-correcting ability would be the case of a person who eats something toxic and immediately vomits. Again, the reaction occurs because the body recognizes a deviation from a state of chemical normality in the stomach and takes immediate steps to restore optimal conditions by removing the source of the problem. From this standpoint, "illness" is simply a manifestation of the body's innate intelligence.

The job of the therapist is to find some way to contact the body's built-in templates of perfection and allow them to blueprint the recovery. This contact can be made in a number of ways. In chiropractic, we begin by making a postural analysis, evaluating the structure of the body with some sophisticated devices, such as a metricon.

This device operates on the principle of converting the contours of the body into electrical impulses, which are then digitized on a computer to give a picture of spinal conformation, rib conformation, or whatever. By turning the patient's head in one direction or another we can measure the degree of rotation. By analyzing structure in this way, we can see what the body has done—and what it is trying to do —in its attempts to conform to its inner ideal blueprint.

For example, in patients with blood-sugar problems (both low and high) we often see a tendency for one shoulder to be higher than the other. The latissimus dorsi is a long muscle that runs from the arm to the pelvis, serving to level the shoulders. When this muscle is weak on one side, the shoulder goes up on that side because the trapezius muscle, which connects the shoulder to the head and neck, pulls it up. Of course, the elevation of one shoulder may represent only a simple musculoskeletal problem; but in many cases the organs that regulate blood sugar—pancreas, small intestine, and liver—are in a state of aberration, and this condition shows up as a tendency for one shoulder to be higher than the other.

We can distinguish between the two cases by a standard of muscle testing, or applied kinesiology, which tells us what the body is trying to do. Body language never lies. Yet body language must be understood here as more than posture or structural alignment, for we know that health depends equally on biochemical and psychological components. So the symbol of applied kinesiology that we use in our form of chiropractic is the equilateral triangle. In this symbol, the base represents structure, one side represents biochemical factors, and the other side represents psychological factors. The whole person, then, exists by way of structure, chemistry, and psychology.

From the standpoint of this threefold model, different schools of healing can be explained by the fact that their practitioners are either structurally, chemically, or psychologically oriented. Those who are structurally oriented emphasize posture and alignment; they practice different forms of bodywork, while tending to deemphasize or ignore the elements of chemistry and psychology. Those who are chemically oriented emphasize pharmaceuticals, herbs, nutrition, and the like, often paying little attention to the elements of structure and psychology. And those who are psychologically oriented focus on methods of working with the mind and emotions—psychotherapy, meditation, shamanism, Christian Science, and so forth.

Of course, it is perfectly natural that those in the healing professions should be inclined to work within the framework of a particular system that is either structurally, chemically, or psychologically based. But one must not let the emphasis of a system blind one to the total picture. One must keep in mind that the structural side of the triangle can affect the chemical and psychological sides, and that, conversely, the chemical and psychological sides can affect the structure. In fact, all sides are interdependent in an equilateral triangle. Unfortunately, however, our mode of living, philosophy, or attitude often makes the triangle isosceles rather than equilateral; that is, we exaggerate the area that our discipline happens to embrace. As a result, we do very well on the long side of the triangle but less well on the short sides.

The obvious solution is to integrate our skills and knowledge in such a way that we gain a full appreciation of the total system as an equilateral triangle. Of necessity, our system has to include structure, chemistry, and psychology. Methods must be used that allow access to all sides of the triangle.

For example, in chiropractic we start from structure but we can gain access to chemistry and psychology from that starting point. By entering through the door of structure and using applied kinesiology, we can discover not only problems requiring physical manipulation but also those requiring nutritional or pharmaceutical agents and those requiring work on aberrant psychological patterns.

Therapists who are mainly structurally oriented need to recognize that patients whose problems can be solved by only physical manipulations are rather scarce. Certainly there are patients whose vertebral structure is slightly compressed on one side or the other, and manipulation of the spine may be all that is necessary to correct the condition. Yet the overly simplistic emphasis on vertebral position that one finds in some schools of healing has not resulted in large numbers of patients cured. Cases in which a difficult chronic condition can be remedied by manipulation alone are the exception rather than the rule. What one generally finds, instead, is the need to take care of chemistry and psychology along with structure. When the diagnostic potential of the structural patterns are refined, as in the kinesiological methods just mentioned, the therapist's ability to deal with a patient's problem is tremendously enhanced.

Also, a patient's chemistry, even his level of hormones, can be influenced by the force of the physician's personality, or "bedside manner." It is no exaggeration to say that many people get better simply because they like the doctor. The positive emotion of "liking" is in itself extremely therapeutic. Laughter, as Norman Cousins demonstrated, is another effective means of stimulating the inner healer.

The personal factor in healing has received far too little attention in Western medicine. Year by year, the health-care system seems to become more and more dehumanized and dehumanizing to the patient, with the result that healers are not able to heal. I find it extremely useful in my own practice to make the patient feel personally involved in the healing process. This I do by analogies, humor, loving care, and especially by intelligent appreciation.

I often say that a doctor should talk like a cracker-barrel philosopher but should also have a razor-edged mind. The trouble is that some practitioners who have sharp minds do not know how to communicate effectively with patients, thereby losing the therapeutic benefits of a personally appealing bedside approach—the virtue of the old family doctor. Of course, sometimes the family doctor lacks the scientific information and technology necessary to deal with a critical problem that is structurally, chemically, or psychologically based. So the true physician must be a man or woman for all seasons, always keeping in mind that whatever method of treatment is adopted, the key is to help the body heal itself. All the therapist has to do is allow the process to occur by removing the impediments.

Brooke Medicine Eagle

THE CIRCLE OF HEALING

Brooke Medicine Eagle, M.A., is a native Earthkeeper, teacher, writer, performer, and celebration leader, as well as a Feldenkrais instructor and a Ropes Course Facilitator. Her visions and teaching have been documented in Shamanic Voices, Shape Shifters, The Spiral Path, *and* The Shaman's Path. *Her forthcoming book,* Buffalo Woman Comes Singing, *will further delineate her earth-centered teachings.*

The origin of the word *heal* gives us a key to the golden thread that unites all methods of healing. *Heal* comes from the same root as *whole* and *holiness,* although this ancient meaning of the word seems to have been forgotten by much of modern Western medicine. I would like to share the teachings about holiness in my own Native American tradition, where holiness and wholeness are still associated with healing.

I often introduce people to the experience of holiness through a simple dance. I invite you to follow along in your imagination as I share it with you.

We gather in a circle, arms around each other's waists, listening as a beating drum echoes the heartbeat of Mother Earth, until the sound resonates within us. Then we each echo the beat by stepping down on the left foot while picking up the right knee, keeping the left foot open and the step deep and gentle on the face of Mother Earth. (If you are sitting as you read this, lean forward and give yourself the physical sense of stepping down with your left foot.)

In doing this we have focused what we call a *first attention*—the attention of our everyday, physical body reality. With it we determine right from left, feel physical weight on one side of the body or the other, step down in rhythm with the drumbeat, feel the presence of others, move with them, and find our balance. For a few moments our entire attention is focused in this basic and primary "Earth dimension" of body consciousness—hence it is called a first attention.

Then we begin moving to the left as we continue to step in time with the drumbeat. (As you read this, try to keep your imagination and body active so that you share the experience rather than just understanding it intellectually.) Now the first attention is engaged even more fully, because the coordination, balance, and rhythm must be more precise as each person on the circle begins moving in rhythm with the others. When we are in a comfortable unity, moving easily with others in the circle, we feel our attention release as the first attention drops into the background of consciousness.

Now I give a *second-attention* task: The dancers are to focus their attention on softening and opening the sole of the left foot, so that they have a growing sense of connection with Mother Earth below. Through the softened and opened sole of the left foot we feel our link with the Earth Mother who supports us in every moment of earthly life, giving us not only food, water, tools, and the materials for shelter, but even the very cells of the bodily temples we inhabit. At this time I say: "Let the heartbeat of Mother Earth—her vibration, her energy, her connection to all other earthly things and beings—fill your body through this open foot."

As the drum continues to beat, I tell the dancers, "Keep bringing your second attention to Mother in acknowledgment, in gratitude. Feel the connection between you strengthen as you open to her and acknowledge her presence in and around you. Mother dances with you. With each step, think of a time when you stepped off that last unexpected stair and felt the nothingness under you. And give thanks to Mother for pushing up under your foot and supporting you."

As the word *Mother* becomes a simple mantra and slips into the background of consciousness, our first and second attentions are integrated. Our third attention awaits.

Now we focus not only on how we are stepping, and not only on Mother Earth, but on the whole circle of dancers. "Feel yourself as a part of one moving unit. Begin to bring your circle into more and more roundness, with no corners or flat places, so that each person can easily see all the others. Notice how each person is both a leader and a follower yet is neither because everyone has the same value on the circle. Notice, too, that each dancer is as slow as the slowest person, as weak as the weakest link."

This attention toward oneness, or wholeness, is what my tradition names *holiness*. As we become whole, holiness extends out, just as we might extend our dance circle metaphorically to include all other human beings. Then, extending further, we might involve all animals, dancing with them as each person calls out the name of one animal and brings it into the circle. Still expanding, we might then contain all growing plants, then all fishes. We dance and bring into the circle all of those who live within and crawl upon Mother Earth. Then we extend it even further, until we include the "star people" and all the universes beyond us, encompassing those who have come before us and those who will come seven generations after us, until finally we embrace All Our Relations, All-That-Is. Such is an act of holiness.

This holiness is the essence of healing, which means to manifest wholeness in spirit and bring it into our bodies, our families, our communities, our world. We heal by beginning to consciously embody the Spirit that lives as one with us and in all things. Thus the function of a healer is to embody and manifest that wholeness of Spirit in such a way that he or she can guide those who have fallen out of rhythm, who have stumbled into dis-ease, and help them to reestablish their balance and rhythm.

Illness is like the momentary feeling we have when we get out of step with the dancing circle. The healer, as impeccable dancer, helps us get back into step with the rhythm of the universe by re-embracing and remanifesting our own wholeness of Spirit.

As we look at the wisdom of the lineages portrayed in this golden thread, we see that Native American medicine people fasted and cleansed themselves for four days. In this way they first became fully aware, present, and alive in their first attention; then by this and other means, such as meditation on the breathing cycle, they came into full second attention and resonance with Mother; until finally they blossomed into the embracing bond of holiness, ready to reflect the spirit of wholeness.

Then a circle would be called together in which the dis-eased one would be laid at the center. The circle might begin by cleansing itself of past history through acts of personal forgiveness; then the dancers might sing songs of harmony and begin to walk in a circle. They would dance an imagined ascending spiral, calling and drawing the descending energy of the patient in the center, until the descent hesitates, stops, and begins to lift upward, carried at first by the community energy but gradually gaining its own strength. At last it would resonate fully within the newly healed one as he or she rejoined the dance. This transformation might take several days and might involve other acts of holiness as well.

In the healing circle, the healer acts as the steady flame of a single candle, awakening with its light the light within all the others, until the flames within the participants burn as one, and wholeness is reflected.

All forms of healing intervention act to disrupt the continuity of the present disorder, the present limiting trance, bringing to bear the deeper resonance of harmony and oneness. An example comes to mind from my own life—picking up a child who is lying on the floor, kicking and crying in great unease, holding him until the storm has passed; and then, perhaps, sharing with him a few dance steps, a few swirls and twirls where our energy resonates and spins, creating laughter as I put the child down to go on his way.

Sometimes when helping a person open to more of the wholeness, extraordinary means are used. These may include fasting, herbal plants, or retreat in a cave. Anything can be used that, without causing damage or unnecessary distress, creates a radical discontinuity in the way the dis-eased person's reality is assembled. Then the dance toward wholeness can begin.

Throughout the process of creating this radical discontinuity, the healer must be able to manifest a larger continuity and harmony within himself or herself, acting as a beacon for the larger circle.

In our everyday world, we are reaching this kind of healing on many levels. We now understand our own health as something created through the pattern of our lives; and we are beginning to understand disease, not as something bad or evil that "comes to get us," but as a symptom of an imbalanced way in which we walk on Mother Earth. With this understanding we can begin the process of healing ourselves through proper nutrition, physical exercise, new beliefs, and a more healthy environment, as well as through the balancing of energies and the right use of medicines that stimulate the body's innate healing capacities.

In this way our healing becomes an accepting, loving expression of all parts of ourselves. We look at the larger whole and understand that polluting this Earth, from which we receive our physical lives, is the beginning of much disease. Thus, by seeing that we are truly one with all things, we see that in supporting the killing of others or the destruction of the natural world, we are inviting that destruction upon ourselves. With this realization we begin the true healing, which means coming into resonance with the Creator's one law: *You shall be in good relationship with each other and with all things in the Great Circle of Life.*

Let us move joyfully in the dance of that larger healing, in the dance of that holy circle.

Part Three

THE HEALER
WITHIN

*The natural healing force within each one of us
is the greatest force in getting well.*

Hippocrates

One of the most fundamental roles a healer can play is to help individuals attune themselves to their own unlimited healing capacities. Each of us has an inner voice or adviser that helps us regulate our internal responses with quiet and truthful guidance. The contributors to this section discuss the importance of creating an environment of support and reflection in which individuals can become receptive to their innate wisdom.

In assisting this process of calling forth our innate wisdom, the healer empowers us to look within for "healing," rather than to external sources for "curing." The healer and the person being healed can then explore the idea that disease may not be a random event; it may be a message telling us that we have deviated from our true path.

The realization that we possess these profound healing powers within us enables us not only to heal ourselves, but also to support others in their healing quests.

John E. Upledger

SELF-DISCOVERY AND SELF-HEALING

*John E. Upledger, D.O., F.A.A.O., D.Sc., has more than twenty years'
experience in the general practice of osteopathic medicine and has been a
member of the faculty at Michigan State University. Through his research
in craniosacral therapy, he has become world-recognized for his diagnosis
and treatment of chronic illness and pain. He heads the Upledger Institute
in Palm Beach Gardens, Florida.*

T he secret something that is shared by all effective healing methods
can perhaps be best characterized as the process of leading the
patient to an honest and truthful self-discovery. This self-discovery is
required for the initiation and continuation of self-healing; for it is
only through self-healing—in contrast to "curing"—that patients can
experience both permanent recovery and spiritual growth.

Before discussing self-discovery and self-healing, however, we
need to examine the meanings of the terms *healing* and *curing.* The
distinction between the two defines a developing polarity in the thinking of health-care professionals. The two words share essentially the
same definition in dictionaries, both referring to a method or course
of remedial treatment that aims to restore health. Yet this official
definition does not capture the implications that the two words have
taken in today's health-care world.

At present we often use the term *healing* to refer to what is done
by the patient (or the patient's body) in order to resolve a problem
of the body, mind, or spirit; whereas the term *curing* usually refers to
what is done *to* the patient by a physician or therapist. So we fre-

quently speak of patients as needing to "heal themselves" after the disease has been "cured." Surgical removal of the gallbladder, for instance, may "cure" gallbladder disease, but the patient must then "heal" the wound and adapt to the absence of that organ in order to achieve adequate function of the digestive system.

The reason we need to clarify the difference between healing and curing is quite simple: Effective therapy—whatever its outer form— initiates, facilitates, and supports the patient's self-healing efforts, whereas the "curing" process is one that provides a more temporary and perhaps only palliative effect. Although "curing" may remove the symptoms of a disease from the outside, so to speak, it usually leaves the underlying causes of the symptoms untouched.

For example, a physician might "cure" hemorrhoids by surgically removing them. If, however, the hemorrhoids are secondary to a congested liver that is due to chronic drinking, the problem will not be "healed" until the patient resolves the underlying reason for the alcohol abuse. In this case, it might be better for the surgeon to leave the hemorrhoids intact, as a reminder and perhaps motivating force that will help focus the patient's attention on the alcohol abuse. In this way the real cause of the problem may one day be eradicated.

A friend and general surgeon with more than thirty years' experience once confided to me that, in retrospect, he felt the majority of surgical procedures he had performed might be classified as excisions of the "vocal apparatuses" of the inner selves of his patients. He meant that by removing certain organs or tissues, he was eliminating the bodily voices that were attempting to communicate the presence of deeper emotional or spiritual problems in need of attention.

Thus, to refer again to our previous example of an alcohol-abusing hemorrhoid patient, we must consider that although removal of the hemorrhoids might temporarily alleviate some of the symptoms, it also removes one avenue by which the inner self is attempting to focus attention on the alcohol problem. If the hemorrhoids are removed and the alcohol abuse continues, the inner self has no choice but to select another organ to use as an attention-getter.

The next "target" organ might be the gallbladder. The next step will be for the surgeon to remove the gallbladder, which may be full of gallstones. Certainly the surgeon feels justified in performing both surgeries, yet no attempt has been made to determine whether the patient's inner self is trying to relay some underlying message to the conscious mind. So we now have a heavily drinking patient without hemorrhoids or gallbladder who still has little or no idea why he or she is abusing alcohol. Perhaps the drinking is a means of escape from guilt feelings instilled during childhood by a parent. If so, the issue is left unexplored and the abuse continues until, eventually, the function of the liver begins to falter.

As the deterioration proceeds, the "inner voice" of the body's wisdom will feel an increasingly urgent need to contact the patient's conscious mind. So it is likely that varicose veins will develop in the esophagus. The situation is now serious and life-threatening, requiring co-management by internal medicine specialists as well as surgeons. Once these veins are surgically dealt with, there is little remaining that can be removed, except the liver itself in the rare cases when a transplant may be undertaken. Usually, however, the internist must support the abused and failing liver until death intervenes.

Let's backtrack a little. Somewhere along the line, a psychiatrist may have been called in to deal with the compulsive alcohol abuse, or because the patient may have been recognized as suicidal. In either case, most of the drugs prescribed by the psychiatrist will probably have both mind-altering and hepatotoxic (liver-poisoning) qualities. Therefore, the "inner voice" will have even less chance of communicating with the drug-compromised conscious mind about the reason for the alcohol abuse (i.e., unresolved guilt), and the liver function will be further impaired by the toxic nature of the drugs. Finally, premature death occurs.

The cause of death will probably be recorded as "liver failure due to alcohol abuse." From our perspective, however, it might be as accurate to say that the cause of death was the hemorrhoidectomy performed without search for an underlying message or cause; or the second excision of the "inner voice," which was attempting to speak through the gallbladder.

Becoming aware of this inner voice is what I mean by the kind of self-discovery that leads to self-healing. In the case just discussed, treatment not only failed to make the patient aware of the inner voice, it ultimately suppressed it. This treatment led to a self-perpetuating cycle of deterioration. Short of a miracle, the process was probably not reversible once the varicose veins developed in the esophagus and the brain was numbed by mind-altering drugs. After all, what chance does the inner voice have against modern surgical technology and psychopharmacology?

In response to the failure of traditional "curing" methods to provide meaningful assistance to those struggling with deeper problems that manifest as body dysfunctions, a myriad of health-related treatment techniques, methods, and philosophies have been created. These include a wide spectrum of practices, such as meditation, nutritional therapy, herbal therapy, homeopathy, acupuncture, Rolfing, chiropractic, Alexander-Feldenkrais technique, rebirthing, counseling, biofeedback, to name a few. Each of these systems, although outwardly different, facilitates the self-discovery that leads to self-healing.

In considering how the process of self-discovery works, it is important to remember that our self-image is constantly changing. It seems that the closer our perception of self approaches the truth, the deeper our capacity for self-healing becomes. When there is a very close correspondence between self-image and truth, our self-healing power may be virtually unlimited, capable of producing the "miracle cure." So, the main responsibility of the therapist is to help the patient develop a truer, more correct self-image.

This means that when working with a patient, the therapist must become an accurate reflecting mirror, a medium through which the patient's real self can be perceived more clearly. This true self-image may not be compatible with the therapist's preconceived notion of the patient's problem, if such a preconceived notion exists. The therapist must become an unbiased facilitator. Then the truth can be discovered by both patient and therapist.

In order to allow for this discovery, the facilitator must remove, as much as possible, the influences of ego and any tendency to engage in diagnostic cataloging. The facilitator can then become a clear reflecting medium that permits no illusion, delusion, camouflage, or facade.

During this process, the facilitator cannot force too much perception of truth at one time or the patient may turn away from the reflection. Therefore, the "mirror" must be very sensitive, reflecting only as much as the patient is able to deal with at any given time. Still, it must reflect enough to prevent stagnation and keep the self-discovery process moving. The art of therapy is in sensing how rapidly the process can move without creating resistance or turning the patient away, and in allowing the patient to make his or her own discoveries. This art requires that the therapist avoid suggestion and leading. It also involves a connection with the patient at an unconscious level. The process of self-discovery may continue with or without words.

My own therapeutic style uses physical touch to facilitate the establishment of a connection between myself and the patient's unconscious. Other therapists may establish this connection by other means, but for me it is the act of touching, of physical contact between myself and the patient, that allows me to establish this communication.

As I blend or merge with the patient by the use of touch, I make every effort to remain open to any perceptions, sensations, or insights that may penetrate into my conscious awareness from the patient. I believe that every organ, tissue, and cell in the body has its own consciousness. This is usually not within the scope of the patient's conscious awareness. However, when I remain open, I receive information from these unconscious parts. These messages may enter my conscious mind as pain in my own body, a visual image, a verbal message, or a sort of knowing or insight that circumvents contributing clues and information fragments along the way.

For example, our patient with the liver problem from alcohol abuse may cause me to experience discomfort in my own liver; or I may see a visual image of a damaged liver; or I may hear the patient's unconscious voice telling me that his liver is damaged; or I may sense that he is a problem drinker due to parent-instilled guilt. When this information is received, my goal is to assist the patient in self-discovery so that he knows that the symptoms are due to alcohol abuse, and why the alcohol abuse came about and why it continues.

The process of communication between patient and therapist is stimulated by the act of touching with intent to assist in the healing process. This patient-therapist communication is initially on an unconscious level. Then it usually emerges into the therapist's conscious awareness. The therapist then works to assist the patient in developing an awareness of the information received. For it is when the patient is consciously informed that he or she can best do something intelligent about the problem. Therefore, in my own practice, I try very hard to reflect a true picture, to be an honest yet sensitive mirror. The patient does not have to see the truth all at once, but I do not aid and abet the continuance of an illusion, unless (as happens in rare cases) it seems very important for the patient to maintain this illusion—and then only for the time necessary for adaption and growth to occur.

When the process of self-discovery has resulted in genuine self-healing, it may or may not produce a "cure"—that is, the elimination of symptoms. For true healing goes deeper than symptoms; it involves getting clear about your real identity and purpose in life. For this reason, healing may sometimes mean spending the rest of your life in a wheelchair—if that is how you can best perform your life task. You may be "healed" even though you remain in a wheelchair, providing you recognize that this is how things are supposed to be for you. Similarly, healing may mean recognizing that it is okay to die. It may mean that the problems and conflicts posed to you for solution during this lifetime have been resolved and that you are now free to leave this environment.

So the successful therapeutic process does not necessarily produce comfort, ease, muscular strength, prolonged life, or any of the other things that our Western medical tradition has come to hold as evidence of healing. Effective therapy does, however, give the individual patient a clear vision of what he or she needs to do, as well as the strength and integration of mind, body, and spirit to do it. The goals of therapy are the elimination of delusion and self-pity and the helping of patients to prioritize and focus their lives so that they can grow.

In the therapeutic process the single most important factor seems to be the ability of the therapist to reflect back the truth to the patient. For it is truth that heals. Truth is the golden thread found in all effective therapeutic systems.

Shakti Gawain

LISTENING TO INNER WISDOM

Shakti Gawain, author of the best-selling books Creative Visualization *and* Living in the Light, *conducts workshops and runs a center in Marin County, California. Her special talent is to help bring spirituality into practical application.*

A healer is someone who helps and supports people in the process of learning to trust their own inner truths and to live more fully and freely. In order to heal themselves, people must recognize, first, that they have an inner guidance deep within and, second, that they can trust it. My own work consists of showing people some simple ways to contact their own deepest wisdom and encouraging them to begin trusting and following it in their lives.

In my view, the root cause of most physical ailments is connected with not living in accordance with one's inner guidance. For the most part, we do not learn how to listen to ourselves. Consequently, we do not trust and take care of ourselves according to what our inner guidance is trying to tell us. We are usually taught to live by certain rules and standards, or to please other people. We must go deeper than these influences if we wish to get in touch with deeper truths.

When we are trying to decide what to do, or when we are not quite certain what we really want, we can usually find the answer just by tuning in to our inner wisdom. This means relaxing beyond the intellect into a deeper place within. Once we can contact that inner guide, we need only ask ourselves, "What feels right to me? What do

I really want? What is true for me at this moment? Where is my energy taking me right now?" With a little bit of practice, most people can learn to do this.

To consider a simple example, suppose you are trying to decide whether to attend a social engagement. If you are like most people, you tend to decide mainly in your mind, by reasoning with yourself: "Well, let's see, if I go to the party, I might meet so-and-so; I might make some good contacts; but maybe it would be better to stay home and rest." Or, you may react from fear: "If I don't go, so-and-so will be offended, and maybe he won't like me; or I might miss something important." This decision making is confined to the realm of ideas.

But if you learn to tune in to your intuition, you will simply have a sense of where the most energy is for you at that moment, and an immediate sense of knowing what you most feel like doing, whether going to the party or staying home or doing something else. This is a mundane illustration, the kind of decision people make all the time; but the principle of listening to one's inner guidance can be applied to more important areas of life as well, such as determining what one's body needs in order to be healed.

I teach people that there are two essential components in the process of tuning in to inner wisdom. The first involves learning some basic skills such as how to relax the body and mind deeply, using simple visualization, breathing, and so forth, so that they can "let go" a little bit. I have them imagine that they are moving into a very deep and quiet inner place where they have a certain wisdom or awareness of what is true for them, and then simply listen or feel what is there. This means asking for an answer and then trusting the reply that comes from that place of inner wisdom.

It is an uncomplicated technique but one that is extremely effective. After my workshops, most people leave feeling that they have made contact with that place inside of them that they can trust. Of course, in our daily lives we do not always feel in touch with this inner guidance; and even if we do, it is sometimes difficult to know exactly what it is trying to tell us. But the more one practices getting in touch with it on a daily basis, the more reliable it becomes.

The second part of what I do involves helping people sort out all the voices and feelings they have inside so that they can distinguish the voice of the real inner guidance. For instance, we may have one inner voice coming from what our mother taught us; another from what our father taught us; others from the influence of our church teachers and friends; and still others from folk heroes and cultural myths. There are voices that tell us what we "should" be doing, and rebellious voices that tell us to do just the opposite.

Because of these conflicting feelings, fears, and desires, it is not enough to say, "Listen to your inner voice." The question is, *which inner voice?*

In my work I use a technique called "voice dialogue," a powerful method invented by Hal Stone and Sidra Winkleman for helping people get in touch with their many different voices, or "subpersonalities," and bring them to conscious awareness. I find that once we do some necessary integrating and balancing of our subpersonalities so that the different inner voices are brought into greater harmony, we discover a deeper awareness of what is best for us in any given moment.

In sorting out these voices, it is important to learn to respect all of them, because those different feelings are there for a reason. We have developed them in an effort to protect and take care of ourselves. A lot of them, however, are outdated and are no longer useful guides. So we must develop our connection with the original, naturally wise being who lives within us and learn to trust our deeper intuitive knowledge.

This, however, does not mean denying or suppressing the other voices. We must come to know, embrace, and accept all of ourselves, including those parts we might consider negative, dark, frightening, or nonspiritual. There has always been this sort of dichotomy between the dark and light, acceptable and unacceptable, good and bad, positive and negative parts of ourselves. We need to recognize that all parts are necessary and important. In fact, the reason things become negative is because we do not accept them or allow them their natural expression.

For example, if we are brought up in an environment that does not allow us to express a natural and creative kind of aggressive impulse, then it gets suppressed, only to come out later in a distorted and destructive form, perhaps through violence toward others or toward ourselves or through emotional or physical ailments. Usually if we trace our negative qualities back to their roots, we find that some important parts of us were denied their natural expression.

An essential part of the process of healing has to do with going into the shadow aspects of ourselves—the aspects that, out of fear, we have denied, disowned, or suppressed. Beginning in a gradual, safe, and comfortable way, we can accept and include them. Then, by allowing them their natural expression, we start to become more fully integrated human beings.

I believe that the healing process going on within us and in the world today has a lot to do with looking into those dark corners and seeing what we have hidden away and have long been afraid to look at. A lot of pain, confusion, fear, and craziness is being flushed to the surface right now. We can see this in the world as well as in our own individual lives. And an enormous amount still must be brought to light and healed through our awareness.

To summarize, then, an effective therapist of any kind is one who can help patients, clients, or students get in touch with inner wisdom and start trusting themselves. Of course, different therapists or healers might express this quite differently. But it seems to me that whenever real healing takes place it is because people find a sense of truth within themselves and learn to trust, honor, and care for themselves in accordance with that truth.

As more therapists and teachers begin to recognize this, healing will become more consciously oriented toward teaching people to trust and take care of themselves rather than to look to outside authorities. In other words, there will be less emphasis on external leaders, healers, and teachers and more emphasis on the empowerment of the individual.

This shift in focus does not mean that there will be no place for teachers, healers, and therapists; it means only that we will increasingly see the roles of teacher and student, healer and patient, changing to a more equal kind of relationship—one in which we will be aware that we are all healing and teaching ourselves and each other.

Another interesting direction that healing is taking has to do with allowing the earth itself to become our teacher and healer. In ancient traditions, the earth and the natural elements were very much our teachers. More recently, we have turned our backs on this earth wisdom and have gone in a different direction, exploring and developing an elaborate technological way of life. But it now appears that the limits of that way of life are being recognized. People are realizing that if we continue on the same course, we are headed for social and ecological disaster.

I think that if we make this turning point successfully and begin listening again to the earth, we will discover that she will teach us how to live in a healthy, balanced, integrated way. Again, the way we can connect with the teaching of the earth and of nature is through our own inner guidance. The more we are able to trust and listen to ourselves, the more we naturally come into balance with all the elements around us. Already we are rediscovering certain ancient traditions that can help us tune in to ourselves and to the earth more effectively. Through cultivation of a greater connection with plants and animals, as well as through music, dance, drumming, and ritual, we are going back to our roots and finding ways to live in greater harmony.

This is the direction in which we need to head, for ultimately we cannot separate the healing of the individual from the healing of the planet. They are one and the same, because the consciousness of each individual is connected to the collective consciousness. Although we are individuals, we are also each a part of the whole. As we begin to heal ourselves as individuals, we also naturally shift the consciousness of the entire planet. And as the collective consciousness begins to shift, we are each in turn affected by it. Thus, the more people change their consciousness and their way of life, the more the world changes; and the more the world changes, the more individuals change.

We are in a profound healing process right now, both individually and collectively. We are on a journey of return to the paradise from which we came as this earth becomes a more healing, nurturing, and beautiful expression of who we really are. Therefore, we can each start to practice listening for our own inner truth, which is deeper than all the various programs, influences, and ideas we have picked up here and there in our lives. Even though our inner guidance may sometimes come to us in the form of those ideas and influences, we need to practice going into the deepest part of ourselves for the sense of what is true and right. If we practice following our inner guidance on a daily basis, asking for advice in the simplest possible way in our lives, we will gradually establish this connection more firmly.

Martin Rossman

ILLNESS AS
AN OPPORTUNITY
FOR HEALING

Martin Rossman, M.D., is founder and director of the Collaborative Medicine Center in Mill Valley, California, a clinical associate in the Department of Medicine at the University of California–San Francisco Medical School, and is a member of the Scientific Advisory Board of the Institute for the Advancement of Health. He is the author of Healing Yourself: A Step-by-Step Program to Better Health through Imagery.

A ll approaches to healing create an opportunity for healing. This may involve the surgical removal of a tumor in order to allow the rest of the body to right itself and take care of whatever pathology remains; or it may mean that a psychotherapist, hypnotist, or shaman creates a situation in which thoughts, emotions, or "spirits" believed to be present in the development of the illness are removed or transformed, allowing the system to reassert its own healthy balance. In each case, creating an opportunity for healing means eliminating those factors that hinder the body's innate capacity for self-healing, and increasing the factors that promote and stimulate that ability.

My own work in preventive medicine and chronic illness is largely based on the premise that healing is a natural occurrence, an innate mechanism of the organism. There is a physiological intelligence that serves to keep the body in homeostasis or balance in the face of all kinds of challenges from both the outer and inner environments.

From this perspective, the symptoms of illness often can be seen as signals for attention or ways of making us aware of needs that are not being met. Thus if we learn to pay attention to our body's signals or symptoms in a certain way, we can actually learn something from an illness that helps to bring us back into alignment with our potential for wellness. For we are always trying to maintain our alignment, balance, and growth in accordance with our purpose in life, whether we are fully conscious of that purpose or not. And there is a way of seeing and relating to symptoms that can actually help us to align the flow of energy in accordance with that purpose—a way that allows us to see illness as an opportunity.

My colleague, Dr. Rachel Naomi Remen, has said that illness could be considered a Western form of meditation. In the West, where the meditative tradition is not strong and people are not in the habit of stopping periodically to become quiet and reevaluate their lives, an illness—and sometimes only a serious illness such as a heart attack or cancer—stops a person so he can step back and have an opportunity to take stock of what is important to him.

In fact, this is a common experience of people with serious illnesses. They often make a profound assessment of their life and values and rededicate themselves to those things of most importance. When a serious illness strikes, people often try to "bargain" with whatever they perceive to be the organizing principle of the universe, saying, "If I recover from this, then I'm going to spend more time with the family," or "I'll develop my creativity," and so forth. Sometimes these promised changes are made, sometimes they aren't; sometimes they last, sometimes they don't. But if there are no changes, or if they are not lasting, the person often gets another "reminder" in the form of a recurrence of illness.

Because of this, I teach a technique called "getting in touch with the inner adviser." This inner adviser might also be called the inner physician or simply one's inner wisdom. In any case, people can gain access to it when they learn to become quiet and receptive. Therefore, I first teach people how to create a state of mental and physical relaxation and calm. In order to help them relax physically, they are shown how to focus their attention on the body, part by part, inviting each part to relax, while at the same time doing deep, full breathing, a process that takes about ten minutes. Then they are asked to imagine themselves in a quiet inner place that is serene and secure. This can be a real or imaginary place. In either case, imagining themselves in this special inner place sets the state for inner dialogue.

I then ask them to allow an image to appear of a very wise, loving figure who knows them well. This is the figure we call the inner adviser. It can appear in virtually any form. Some people see archetypal figures such as the Wise Old Man or Wise Old Woman. Others visualize lights, spirits, power animals, trees, or even the ocean. The form does not matter as long as it represents something wise and loving that knows them well. After this, I encourage them to ask the inner adviser if it knows anything about the illness they are experiencing, if there is anything they can learn from it, and if there is anything they can do to help them recover. I encourage them to be open and receptive to the inner adviser's message.

What comes back is often surprisingly relevant. It usually consists of simple yet accurate and frequently elegant advice. This may address physical changes, such as modification of diet, or emotional and spiritual adjustments, such as the resolution of inner conflicts that may be necessary in order to allow the system to come back into balance. The technique is a way of turning the challenge and difficulty of an illness into an opportunity to learn something that can help the person move toward a higher level of wellness.

I frequently use a related technique called "listening to your symptom." This consists of focusing on a symptom, allowing an image to represent it, and then engaging the image of the symptom in dialogue in order to find out why it is there, what it wants, and how you can meet the needs it represents.

Most of the people I see in my practice find these two techniques useful. And over the years I have observed a great increase in the number of people who approach health and illness in this manner. Many people now, for example, come to me describing some symptom and saying, "I feel like my body is trying to tell me something, but I don't know what."

But most people still feel dissociated from the body and tend to perceive illness as something that just happens at random. Such people think of going to a doctor like taking their car to a mechanic: Something is broken and needs fixing. To them, the idea that the body may be intelligent, that it may be sending meaningful signals for the purpose of helping to bring the body back into balance, is something radically new. Sometimes it takes a serious illness to get them started on this type of thinking.

In short, illness can create a situation that demands we evaluate how we are taking care of ourselves, where we are going in life, and what is most important to us. Paying attention to the early warning signals of illness—that is, not waiting until the symptoms become serious, but regarding more subtle symptoms with respect—can often be preventive. Better yet, simply taking regular time to become relaxed and quiet in order to evaluate one's life on an ongoing basis can even eliminate the need to experience illness.

If we regard symptoms as intelligent messages intended to help us reestablish a healthy balance, then when symptoms appear, the important questions to ask are: What is needed here? What can we do to support the self-healing ability of the body and mind? And what should we *not* do that might hinder that ability? Learning to listen to our own inner wisdom can help us develop this awareness.

Clearly, the more knowledge and self-awareness you have, the more able you will be to support the process of reestablishing a healthy balance. And it is here, in this development of greater knowledge and self-awareness, that the physician/therapist/healer can play an important role—a role that may be catalytic and supportive to the person's innate healing faculties. This is true whether the healer is a shaman, a psychotherapist, or a surgeon.

Perhaps the most important thing I have learned from my work is that I can be a friend and supporter of healing; I can be a guide to people; but it is not *I* who does the healing. I try to help create situations that seem to allow or foster healing—calmness, faith, belief, hope, enthusiasm—and sometimes just the idea that healing is a possibility. I attempt to help the person engage with his or her own healing potential and hope that the larger power that gives us both life will bring healing.

One of the major occupational hazards of the healing arts is an overidentification with the ability to heal. Therapists need to keep in mind that their healing ability consists mainly of a gift for influencing, stimulating, and inspiring clients to move along the course of their own healing path; and sometimes nothing the therapist does will work.

This is the second common denominator that stands out in all healing modalities: None of them works all the time. We don't know why. Yet, even in terminal situations, healing can take place, even though it is not physical. Deep emotional and spiritual healing can accompany fatal illness as well as recovery, and we can learn to be a friend to that as well.

Part Four

THE HEALING
RELATIONSHIP

---

*Medicine is not only a science,
but also the art of letting our own individuality
interact with the individuality of the patient.*
                    Albert Schweitzer

The quality of the healing relationship rather than the technique may be the hidden foundation for healing. In this section, the contributors discuss the magic and beauty that occur when two people join to bring forth the healing potentials of healer and the person healed. It is this special bond, created from compassion, trust, and the willingness to move forward together, that transforms the process from curing to healing.

From the joining of hearts and minds comes the realization that we are indeed one in our suffering. In the presence of this relationship, both healer and client explore the depth of their experiences and resources. It is through this unity that both parties can indeed be healed.

Norman Cousins

THE HEALING EQUATION

Norman Cousins, Ph.D., is chairman of the Task Force in Psycho-neuroimmunology and adjunct professor of medical humanities in the School of Medicine at UCLA. He is also the author of twenty popular books, including Anatomy of an Illness, The Healing Heart, Human Options, The Physician in Literature, *and, most recently,* The Human Adventure *and* Pathology of Power.

Healing can be regarded as an equation. On one side of this equation are the resources of medical science together with the body's own healing system. On the other side are the forces that generate or contribute to disease.

Variables outnumber constants on both sides of the equation. Medical science and our knowledge of the factors involved in disease are far from complete. So is our knowledge of how the body's own healing system works. However, we do know that the healing system involves not just a single organ but the totality of all the body's systems.

The "healing system" is not treated as such in medical textbooks; it's not listed in the index along with the digestive system, the circulatory system, or the autonomic nervous system. The healing system is said to be just another term for the immune system. Yet the immune system does not repair a broken bone or close a wound, even though it attempts to combat infections resulting from such events. The healing system involves this protective mechanism, but it also superintends everything involved in restoration and repair. For example, when a fingernail is cut, a signal goes out to the brain, which sends an increased supply of porcelain-type cells to the area of the injury. These cells are converted into fingernail, at which point another signal tells the brain that extra porcelain-type cells are no longer required. If the nail is cut again, the process starts all over.

The human body is a composite manufacturing plant superior to anything known in industry or technology. In addition to porcelain, it can manufacture analogues of wood, silk, plastic, and prisms, among other substances—and all this in factories that are microscopic in size —on location as needed. Not much is known about the process by which this on-site conversion takes place, except that it is complex and amazingly efficient. We live on casual terms with our bodily wonders, hardly pausing to reflect on their presence or how they operate.

The complex interactions between the brain, the endocrine system, and the immune system are perhaps the most explicitly involved components of the body's healing system. The brain is both the seat of consciousness and a gland—perhaps the most prolific gland in the human body. The secretions produced by the brain help to reduce pain and activate biological forces that can combat invaders, stimulate the production of enzymes and other chemical substances, and increase the number of disease-fighting immune cells. Some immune cells, for example, have the capacity to "pry open" cancer cells and deposit the body's own chemical poisons, killing off the cancer cells one by one. All these variables must be included in the healing equation.

Certain variables, of course, can affect the ability of the body to mobilize against disease. Under circumstances of depression, anxiety, or panic, for example, the function of the immune system may be impaired, as indeed are other bodily systems. However, once the patient is liberated from such negative emotions or experiences, the immune system often responds at a higher level.

Attitudes and emotions, therefore, play an obvious and verifiable role in the healing process. Positive emotional factors such as a strong will to live, blazing determination, a sense of purpose, and a sense of festivity may be regarded as blockers against the negative factors that tend to pull down the immune system. In a sense, then, the positive emotions are involved in the war against disease. It is not only the negative attitudes and emotions that affect health; the body is a reciprocal mechanism. Everything that affects it emotionally has an impact, for good or ill.

Positive attitudes and emotions can enhance the environment of effective medical care. Patients who have confidence in themselves and their physicians may be better able to make use of medical treatment than those who go into treatment with attitudes of despair or defeat. Obviously, positive attitudes are not a substitute for medical treatment but an integral part of it. One thing I have learned is that attitudes should not be underestimated in any assessment of the healing equation.

Although I am not an M.D., I have worked with and observed more than five hundred patients during my ten years at the UCLA Medical School. It seems clear to me that few things are more important than the way the physician communicates with the patient. I cannot think of a single case in which reassurance of the patient is not required or justified. Unless the possibility of something good is attached to the prospect of treatment, the environment of treatment may be impaired. Attitudes about treatment can have an effect on the immune system. The patient's hopes are the physician's best ally. The physician who works with those hopes and bolsters them helps to create a climate in which the "little black bag" can be put to optimal use.

Conversely, if a patient comes away from a diagnosis in a state of emotional devastation, the stage may be set for rapid advance of the disease. Despair can damage the environment of effective medical care. Dealing with the patient's attitudes calls for a great deal of artistry. This does not imply that the physician should deceive the patient. A truthful diagnosis must be given, but the physician's artistry consists of an ability to communicate a diagnosis as a challenge rather than as a pronouncement of doom.

I admire physicians who can present a patient with a catastrophic diagnosis, yet do so in a way that brings out the best in the patient. No one should ever leave a doctor's office without hope. The wise physician recognizes that the medical journals regularly carry accounts of remissions that run counter to the predictions of the experts. The accounts of these remissions can be therapeutic, for they can raise the patient's hopes to a higher plateau. That is why the wise physician will mobilize every possible medical resource, as well as help the patient to mobilize his own resources—namely, the body's own healing system.

In the healing equation, therefore, the physician brings the best that medical science has to offer, and the patient brings the best that millions of years of evolution have to offer. But the physician's "best" does not consist solely of technology; an essential ingredient is the way in which the patient's belief system is involved and put to work. The physician who leaves the patient only with negative thoughts sets the stage for panic and depression, thus reducing even further the patient's chance to make optimal use of treatment.

Too many patients have refuted the melancholy predictions of physicians to warrant grim forecasts. It is fair to say the physician is never justified in giving up on any case, or in saying or doing anything that weakens the patient's determination to do his or her own part of the job. Although we ought never to underestimate the seriousness of a medical problem, it is equally important never to underestimate the ability of the patient to mount a prodigious response to the challenge of disease.

No one wants to give patients false hopes; neither do we want to give them false fears. Unfortunately, physicians' lawyers often advise their clients to tell patients the worst as a strategy for avoiding malpractice suits. But the trouble with telling patients the worst is that it has a tendency to bring on the worst. In the realm of healing, we tend to move along the path of our expectations.

This fact points again to the need for artistry. No doubt doctors must seek to protect themselves against malpractice suits. But statistics show that those physicians who are closest to their patients are the ones who are sued the least. A good relationship between patient and physician is perhaps the physician's most powerful tool for dispelling panic and mobilizing the patient's body to exert its maximum force against disease. The concept of a patient-physician partnership is perhaps the strongest such factor in the healing equation.

Rachel Naomi Remen

THE SEARCH FOR HEALING

Rachel Naomi Remen, M.D., F.A.A.P., is in the private practice of behavioral medicine in Sausalito, California, specializing in chronic and life-threatening illness. She is medical director of the Commonwealth Cancer Help Program and serves on the Scientific Advisory Board of the Institute for the Advancement of Health and the Institute of Noetic Sciences.

A healing technique is a vehicle for connecting with another person in a certain way that promotes the movement toward wholeness. Each of us has a technique—perhaps several—that has to do, in some way, with our personality. In my own case, for example, imagery is a powerful technique. I tend to think in images. Other people choose other techniques according to their personal preferences. But the essence of their work remains the same.

A technique is a way of expressing something. The technique is not the healing; it is a vehicle for the healing. We have to ask, beyond all these techniques, what it is that truly fosters the healing process. I think it is the way we stand in relationship to each other that is most important.

When you're working with someone in a healing relationship, something that's never been there before—a wholeness—will start to emerge. The relationship has to be spacious enough, flexible enough, so that this emerging wholeness isn't closed down or interpreted in too hurried a fashion.

I like the archetype of the Wounded Healer, which symbolizes that two people in a healing relationship are peers, both wounded and both with healing capacity. Just by being here, in these bodies, we are wounded, we are incomplete, if you will. But we also have the capacity for wholeness as part of our birthright. It comes out of our human nature. If you and I are participating in the healing process together, it is my woundedness that allows me to connect to you in your woundedness. I know what suffering is. I also know that you may feel separated from other people by your suffering. You may feel lost, frightened, trapped. My woundedness allows me to find you and be with you in a way that is nonjudgmental. You are not the sick one or the weak one. We are here together, both capable of suffering, both capable of healing.

My very presence facilitates something. I sit with you, and you don't have to be alone in this small, dark, fearful place in yourself. You sense that you can trust me. I, too, am wounded, so I can understand. I know how to find you and be there with you, not to "fix" anything—because nothing may be broken—but simply to be there with you in that place where you thought you could only be alone. If we do that, something happens. The woundedness in each of us connects us in trust. My woundedness evokes your healer, and your woundedness evokes my healer. Then the two healers can collaborate together. My presence with you allows things to change, to evolve toward wholeness.

In a true healing relationship, both heal and both are healed. When only one person is seen as the healer, the relationship might be said to be a curing relationship but not a healing one. Often the person who identifies himself as the curer or fixer-type healer is vulnerable to burnout. The curing relationship is not always healthy for the client. While benefiting in some ways by the relationship, the client may also be diminished because it is a dependent relationship. There is not much room for strength or growth in the kind of curing relationship that we're taught in professional schools. We can fix the fixable, but we don't evoke healing, and we don't participate in the healing that may arise naturally. The fixing relationship assumes that healing is not natural. Healing *is* natural. We need to find a way to remind each other of this.

I don't believe that one person heals another. I believe that what we do is invite the other person into a healing relationship. We heal together. Even defining a person as a healer seems to assume some sort of fixing or repairing. A better definition would be inviting someone to participate in life with us, to participate in that movement toward wholeness that underlies all life.

Years ago, I was invited to a seminar given by Carl Rogers. I had never read his work, but I knew that the seminar, attended by a group of therapists, was about "unconditional positive regard." At the time, I was highly skeptical about this idea, but I attended the seminar anyway. I left it transformed.

Rogers's theories arose out of his practice, and his practice was intuitive and natural to him. In the seminar, he tried to analyze what he was doing for us as he did it. He wanted to give a demonstration of unconditional positive regard in a therapeutic session. One of the therapists volunteered to serve as the subject. As Rogers turned to the volunteer and was about to start the session, he suddenly pulled himself up, turned back to us, and said, "I realize there's something I do before I start a session. I let myself know that I am enough. Not perfect. Perfect wouldn't be enough. But that I am human, and that is enough. There is nothing this man can say or do or feel that I can't feel in myself. I can be with him. I am enough."

I was stunned by this. It felt as if some old wound in me, some fear of not being good enough, had come to an end. I knew, inside myself, that what he had said was absolutely true: I am not perfect, but I am enough. Knowing that, at some deep level, allows healing to happen.

I don't self-criticize my work with clients. I simply do what I do and trust what will happen. At the end of a series of sessions, I try to get feedback from my clients. I need to know what is working for people and what isn't. One of the first times I did this was with a powerful woman lawyer. During the last session, I said to her very formally, "I thought it would be good for us to review what has happened here."

"That would be wonderful," she said.

"Grand," I said. "I'd like to ask you, did you get what you came for?"

She replied, "Absolutely not."

I was flabbergasted. I asked what she meant.

She said, "Rachel, when I came here I didn't know that what I got even existed."

It seems to me that's an important dimension of healing. When the wholeness emerges, it is a surprise. It is beyond the mind's conception. Our minds want to fix everything. The wholeness is so much more than that. The healing relationship needs to be unstructured enough to allow that wholeness to emerge. Being present and waiting —almost like waiting for a birth—is an important part of this; so is the concept of not deciding ahead of time what will be needed.

When I was originally trained in pediatrics, the method was simple and straightforward: You walked in, made a diagnosis, decided what was needed, and provided it. The focus was on what *you* as the physician thought, perceived, and decided—a very lonely business. That's the standard medical disease model.

Since then, I've discovered that basically I don't know what's needed. But if I listen to the client, to the essential self of the other person—the soul, if you like—I find that at the deepest level of the unconscious mind, the client knows what's needed. If I can be present at that moment, without having any expectations of what the client is supposed to do, how he or she is supposed to change in order to be "better," what happens is magical. By that I mean it has a deep sense of integrity about it, much more than any diagnosis I could make on my own or any therapeutic strategy I might devise.

Aldous Huxley writes in *The Perennial Philosophy* that all religions share certain commonalities which, if they were understood, might define the nature of God. I like to think of these universal beliefs as the footprints of God. If we examine all the healing systems, we could in the same way find commonalities that might help us come closer to the footprints of healing.

There seem to be certain universal conditions that encourage the movement toward wholeness on a physical level, others on an emotional level, still others on a mental level, and lastly some on a spiritual level. These are probably the same for every human being everywhere and derive from our common human nature, our basic human needs. There are also other more personal conditions of healing that come out of our own unique natures. We need to study the universal conditions as well as the personal conditions that encourage our own healing.

One of these universal conditions seems to be that healing is facilitated when more than one person is concerned. There's a kind of critical mass of consciousness that promotes the healing process. The person who feels isolated and separated is vulnerable. For the person who is connected in a caring and concerned relationship, healing is facilitated. Just knowing that one's well-being matters to somebody else seems to make healing easier, more accessible, more possible.

Personal conditions of healing can be quite varied. Some people get well because they have work to do. Others get well because they feel they've been released from their work and the pressures and expectations of other people. Some people need music; others need to enjoy nature. Many different things remind us of our healing capacity and evoke it.

The study of healing systems may show us that certain kinds of relationships promote healing. I think there's also a certain attitude toward one's self that can promote healing.

Living in one piece is important for healing—in other words, knowing what your deepest values are and living by them, so that there is a coherence between who you are and how you live. If you believe one way but live another, that can be more damaging than any external stress. When you become separated from your own sense of values, it is very hard to heal.

You may have lived by another person's values all your life and not have known it. It may be that you adopted those values when you were very young. But they're still not your own. That is an enormous drain on vitality. In illness, sometimes, people go back to their original values, even though they've never lived by them before. And, in that process, their healing is facilitated.

I don't have any great theories about my clients, or strategies. I simply meet with them and be there with them. I am often asked what happens in my sessions with clients. To tell the truth, I can't answer that. I don't know ahead of time what I'm going to do in a session. I have no plan. But I know that something will happen, and it's not random. I sit with this other person and together we connect to the edge of what we're weaving together, and we weave it a little further along. The energy is always there—I trust that. It's always there, but it's in the relationship, not in me.

I once had an experience that illustrates what I'm trying to say. A psychiatric resident from a nearby hospital told me he wanted to learn how to work with people with cancer. I said he could sit in on some of my sessions. Of course, only some of my clients were willing to have him there. He would sit in the corner, making profuse notes.

After the first session, he said to me, "That was an incredible session. Look, I have the whole thing here." He laid on the floor three pieces of paper covered with notes and lines, like an algorithm in which he had traced the choice points and the entire path of the session. He asked me, "Is this right?"

I replied, "I have absolutely no idea. I don't think I could have created that outline. In fact, I know I couldn't have."

"Well," he asked, "what were you doing? How did you know to go this way or that?"

I said, "I was just following the energy."

"What do you mean by that?"

"I can't tell you," I answered. "I just went in the natural direction of the energy and I could feel it. It's almost like there's a knot of energy in the room and we just keep talking together and working and dancing and singing until that knot begins to loosen, and we are free."

From my point of view, that's all there is to it. I used to be ashamed of not being able to provide a cognitive framework or justification for my interventions. I don't feel that way anymore.

Healing is natural. It's not magical; it's not mystical. It doesn't require some esoteric intervention. It's your birthright, and mine. Everybody has the capacity for healing. We do it with each other all the time and we don't even know it.

Healing is the very ground of being. Everything is moving toward wholeness. And that's all healing is, that movement. Our task is not to make something happen but to uncover what is already happening in us and in others, and to recognize and foster those conditions that nurture it. That's all.

We can do that with ritual or prayer, or with many different approaches and techniques. We can simply sit and be together and think about our true nature. No one technique is inherently any better than another. It's simply a matter of learning to trust the natural healing process in all of us and moving freely with it.

I, for one, am rather taken aback with talk of certain people being "healers." In my opinion, this just separates people from the naturalness of their own healing. And that's the magical thing, that ordinariness, because the ordinary is the most extraordinary thing of all.

Emilie Conrad-Da'oud

TEACHING
WHAT I LIVE

Emilie Conrad-Da'oud is the originator of Continuum Movement, based in Los Angeles, which has broken new ground in the awareness of movement. She applies her work to people who have paralysis and other physical disorders.

When people come to me with an illness or a vital issue troubling them, I agree to collaborate with them. What I mean by collaborate is that I use my experience to observe, listen, offer suggestions, and generally move with the person in a kind of dance. It's a *pas de deux* in which we explore what is unfolding.

After all, healing is mainly a matter of paying attention to the moment, and whatever is going to illuminate the moment is something that can't be decided in advance. It can't be made an intention. All I can do is be there—open, listening, sensing. When someone feels honored and respected in his own particular movement, he enhances his access to his own creative healing possibilities. It's as if each person is reaching into a core of health, a core of sanity.

It's not the method of healing that matters. Clinging to a method imprisons the facilitator. Too many therapists are preoccupied with procedures, not knowing that they themselves *are* the method. The degree to which you can enrich your own perceptions is the degree of your real helpfulness to someone else. I see the method as simply a means, like a surfboard; you ride the healing waves with it.

These waves are something subtle inside us, a trust that takes place in the heart. When people can really trust, when they are able to let go of their feelings of isolation and abandonment, they begin to communicate with their bodies and to address their disease. The difficulty, from a therapist's point of view, is that trust has no particular form to it. It doesn't matter what the technique is. It depends on something the client senses in the quality of engagement itself. When there is trust, the client feels the echo, feels himself in the therapist. And this trust becomes the seed from which the healing process can grow.

At a time of great trauma in my life, I went to see a therapist. I don't think he had a specific therapeutic method; he simply came into my world. He could feel where I was, and he flew parallel with me. He recognized what was going on with me and treasured it. It felt like a flight into sanity. He knew that I was going through a creative crisis, and he knew how to draw out the creative spark that was emerging. From that experience I know that when you do not feel alone, when someone is there with you, magic happens.

People have a real need to express their creativity, to have their creative potential honored. At times we may not allow the creative intelligence of the client to be the primary resource for what is taking place in healing, because we ourselves do not trust the transitional state. In that instance, we may harm the gentle bud of the creative spark. I see creativity as an ocean, a flow, the water we swim in. It is the source of the waves that heal.

One of the keys to healing is to view the whole organism as movement. Everything in the world is moving. Movement is a way of sensing the world as an organism, feeling it at a visceral level or even deeper, at a cellular level. Unfortunately, most people live in a state of fragmentation in which they think in terms of mind and body, inside and outside, up and down.

In movement, particularly at the cellular level, there are no categories. It's our mental framework that creates the boundaries. We learn to create them through what I call consensus. Society constantly regulates itself through common opinion. This social consensus tends to see things not as a whole but as fragments. It divides things into pieces artificially and then acts as if the boundaries are real. It's this thinking process, the way people have compartmentalized the world, that traps their energy and their sense of movement and keeps them from understanding what their fullness can be.

For people to experience themselves as movement is one of the most important perceptions they can have about the world. That means no longer thinking of body/mind, inside/outside, physical/

spiritual, but seeing instead that a person is actually a nexus of many kinds of movements happening together, movements that are flowing and affecting each other. Movement and being human mean the same thing. Every confluence, every conflict in this universe is in us.

I live my life in terms of my sense of movement. I don't structure it too much. I allow for a lot of open time so that I can move with whatever I need to do at that moment. In a sense, I am always in the water; the way I move, the way I teach, the way I do anything—they are all one creative thing. I am not teaching according to method. I am teaching what I live.

Jerry Solfvin

THE HEALING RELATIONSHIP

Jerry Solfvin, Ph.D., teaches parapsychology at the Graduate School of Human Consciousness at John F. Kennedy University in Orinda, California. He has coauthored several books, including Research in Parapsychology 1984 *(with Rhea White) and* Psychic Science and Belief of Man *(with Stanley Krippner).*

F or some time I have been convinced that the common denominator, the golden thread that runs through all forms of healing, may be called the healing relationship. Actually, the healing relationship is not a single factor. Most of us, as children, experienced a healing relationship with our parents. With their kisses they eased the pains of childhood bumps and scrapes and wounded feelings. Some of us were fortunate enough to have had a healing relationship of a different sort with another adult as well, perhaps a grandparent or a favorite uncle or aunt. And, of course, there were the siblings who saw us as no one else ever would, for better or for worse. These family bonds are the cornerstone of our later healing relationships.

Growing older, we may have had a special friend who made us feel that everything was okay. Teachers or neighbors helped soothe the more complex wounds of adolescence. In the teenage years, most of us begin to experience a healing relationship with a group beyond our family. We have teams, clubs, and gangs to heal our longing for a sense of self. At this time, too, many of us begin a healing relationship with God. At some point, romantic healing bonds are formed and we learn new ways to hurt, new ways to heal.

An especially important healing relationship is formed in marriage. For many of us, it is the first time we truly take on the responsibility of the healer. It is often our first voluntary commitment to another human being. It may be the first time that we work truly as a team, that we let down our boundaries and allow ourselves to penetrate and be penetrated by another person. In an intimate relationship, our powers and weaknesses are laid bare. We learn new ways to say "help me," and we listen for our partner's cry. At times we are pressed to the limits of our endurance, unable to make or hear another cry for help. The healing relationship is not always healthy. Some make it through, others do not.

The quality and quantity of these healing relationships help to lay the groundwork for others as we progress through life. Healing relationships are important to our development because they may provide the key that unlocks the virtually limitless self-healing abilities that are our natural potential. With the current interest in self-healing and in the wonders of the immune and regenerative systems, we have only begun to scratch the surface of this latent healing force. I take all stories of miraculous healings, spontaneous remissions, and instantaneous cures as evidence for the remarkable self-healing abilities that are possible in all humanity.

A good place to observe this self-healing ability in action is among our fellow mammals in the wild. A few years ago, while visiting the Gilgil Baboon Project in Kenya, I heard the following anecdote from ethologists at the site. One of the baboons in the colony under observation was swinging on the high-tension wires that cross through their territory when a bare strip of wire touched her head and blew off half of her skull. Although she regained consciousness, the crew concluded that death was certain because her brain was exposed to infection and damage. Remarkably, she didn't die. Skin soon grew to reseal the cranium, and within a few months the baboon was back to normal. Such a wound in a human would certainly be considered fatal without medical intervention. Perhaps we have lost touch with just how powerful the self-healing mechanisms can be.

It is not hard to imagine how people living in urban, industrialized settings may have lost touch with their inner healing mechanisms. For one thing, modern society has hypnotized us into the belief that we need medical intervention in order to heal. It is estimated that 75 to 95 percent of the patients in America who come to hospitals and clinics for treatment have minor, self-limiting disorders that would heal themselves in a few days or weeks. Yet we flock to healers with the hope and expectation of being fixed by them. We are brought up to believe that our diseases must be treated, perhaps by some new wonder drug, to return us to health. Few among us are strong enough to resist this societal belief.

Secondly, modern society creates much of the disease that inflicts us. We sit long hours in front of computers and TV sets, work and live in concrete and metal structures with little sun or fresh air, eat artificial foods, breathe noxious fumes indoors and out, wear clothing that binds our blood flow or denies needed ventilation to parts of our bodies. Moreover, the pace and pressures of modern society build stress and tension that we are only now learning how to deal with. The diseases created by this way of life are difficult challenges for our self-healing abilities. The immune system can deal with stress, but how long can it continue to do so if the stressors are not reduced? We are, in essence, turning our own immune systems against us. In the process, we are losing sight of their incredible powers to heal our bodies and minds.

The healing relationship is important because it holds the potential for reacquainting us with our own self-healing abilities. It is a special form of communication that restores our faith in the so-called miraculous, just as our parents taught us through their comforting kiss how quickly wounds can heal. The healing relationship communicates the love and concern of others that gives us strength and reason to heal. It communicates our worth as an individual. It communicates the irrational, just as love is irrational, and gives us hope that everything is possible through love. The healing relationship communicates high expectations for ourselves, our bodies, minds, and spirits, and motivates us to respect ourselves.

The healing relationship is potentially present whenever one person comes to another for healing. Regardless of the diagnosis or prescription, the healing relationship is a tool all healers can use, and excellent healers throughout the ages have always used it. It encompasses the Hippocratic ideal of setting the stage for healing to take place. It is invoked by the magical rituals of shamans and by the psychotherapist. It is not restricted to licensed healers, but can be invoked by all persons through their love and caring for another human being.

A particularly poignant example of the healing relationship was noted recently in a laboratory study in which rabbits with kidney disorders were being used to test a new drug treatment. When the results were tallied, it was found that, quite separate from the main hypothesis, the rabbits attended by one particular lab technician showed remarkable improvements in their conditions regardless of whether they were given the new drug or a control. When questioned, the technician said that he had handled his rabbits extensively, loving each and every one. The other technicians had not done this. The researchers repeated the study, this time asking half of the technicians to "love" their rabbits, and asking the other half not to do so. The results confirmed the earlier finding: The "loved" rabbits were much healthier.

Human beings living in modern industrialized societies are not so different from caged rabbits. Our environments have decreased the natural self-healing abilities that our wild brothers have retained. The potential may still be there, however, and we need that special something extra to release it. We need the healing relationship—the loving touch, the positive expectancy, the sense of self-worth, even a bit of magic. Healers in all traditions hold the power to evoke this healing relationship. It is the golden thread of healing.

Ted Kaptchuk

HEALING AS A
JOURNEY TOGETHER

Ted Kaptchuk, O.M.D., is clinical director of the Pain and Stress Relief Clinic at Boston's Lemuel Shattuck Hospital. He has a doctorate in Oriental medicine and is one of the few alternative healers who work in conventional hospital settings. His first book, The Web That Has No Weaver, *is considered a classic treatise on Chinese medicine.*

P ractitioners of different medical traditions have various strategies to address the discomforts and disabilities of life. Sometimes their techniques can create change, sometimes they cannot. Each tradition or healing modality has its own set of definitions, categories, and tools for intervention. Surgeons remove tumors, acupuncturists balance *qi,* shamans placate demons or remove spiritual intrusions, chiropractors adjust spinal misalignments, internists supply deficient hormones, psychologists release repressed emotions, and faith healers connect clients to the forces of will and belief. Each practitioner, whatever the technique, has his or her own ideas of what is important in the cosmos and what is the most effective catalyst for change.

There is no question that the techniques of any given medical system are important. They are the cornerstones. But they have an inherent limitation. Each approach reduces the complexity of the person, who is a unique being, into some category that can be understood and manipulated. Stephanus, a sixth-century Greek doctor of Byzantium, understood this dilemma implicitly when he said that medicine suffers from a fundamental contradiction: its theory grasps universals only, while its practice deals with individuals. Because no two people are alike, the differences are ineffable and cannot be subjected to concepts.

How, then, is the gap between a medical technique and a particular individual effectively bridged? How can we get beyond the ideological stance of a medical system? How does a practitioner of a particular strategy still manage to touch another human being, deeply and in a very personal way? Is there a common thread shared by the healing arts that allows the ineffable to be embraced? I believe there is.

Socrates, in a Platonic dialogue, tells young Charmides in the gymnasium of Taureas that he knows of an herb that relieves headache, but that it only works when it is taken with a "charm." This universal charm, it seems to me, has to do with a resonance between the healer and patient that captures the ineffable.

The poetry of this charm evokes understanding and a sense of connection. The charm is forged in a special ritual of trust, intimacy, responsibility, reliance, and care that underlies all healing. The healer's concern, attention, and love for the patient serve to create a special bond, thus moving a simple medical treatment into the realm of a healing art.

The self-conscious healer is not interested in cure alone but rather in healing. The healer knows the true path into the core of a disorder. Genuine healing is a journey, facilitated by a healer, into a broken and hurt self, the purpose of which is to encounter a depth of humanity deeper than the tragedy of any illness. The healer takes a person into the disorder and brokenness, whether it is curable or incurable, to find an intactness and reconciliation that profoundly reflects and manifests the genuine self.

Healing is a crucible to encounter the source of our being in our worst times; it is our genuine and potentially intact response to chaos, anguish, and suffering. Healers forge the illness, the techniques, and their special healing relationship into an opportunity to uncover the truth of who we really are.

Healing is not something we do only when we are sick; it is part of the process and journey of life.

Rosalyn Bruyere

THE COMPASSION FACTOR

Rosalyn Bruyere is founder of the Healing Light Center Church in Glendale, California. She teaches and lectures around the world on "laying on of hands" healing. She has been closely associated with research projects on healing at UCLA and is author of the forthcoming book, Wheels of Light.

Healing arises out of compassion. Compassion is a genuine concern for the pain of another. It is distinct from empathy, which requires identification with another and cannot be linked to one's own search for enlightenment. Compassion reflects a desire for the surcease of someone's sorrow, no matter the differences or similarities between healer and patient. Without compassion, the healer lacks the will to seek an answer, to research the problem, determine a treatment form, and follow through in what may be an arduous struggle to awaken the soul of the sufferer.

The healer uses ritual to create a focus of attention, to move out of the personal into the transpersonal, and trigger or reinforce the compassionate response. The healer establishes a sacred space, or *temenos,* cut off from the ordinary, in which energy can be generated. In the ancient world, and among more primary (as opposed to primitive) cultures in our own time, the existence of sacred or holy places was and is understood. A mountain is a sacred place because a unique magnetic field exists there. In the absence of such a natural field, the healer claims one, in order to create a kind of accelerator or accumulator in which change and growth are quickened. This timeless, suspended place, where there is more harmony and less pain, may also entice the patient's soul, without which there is no real healing.

Ancients and moderns alike complain of suffering as a soulless state. Part of the role of ritual is to coax the soul into participating in a time of need. In some religions, this means coaxing God. Others view it as inviting an aspect of the human soul that does not reside in temporal lives. The compassionate healer, whose soul is present, awakens the other's soul.

This mergence of souls is an experience of hugeness, and of "single-celledness." For the healer who has felt it, each occurrence carries intense relief, a brief respite from the loneliness of experiencing oneself as separate. There is a unique understanding of one's role in the act of healing, and an assurance that one is not working alone but has a connection with the rightness and power of the universe. Out of this connection, compassion is renewed and deepened. It is from this well, from the change that this experience creates in the healer, that compassion for the next being in pain will spring.

Whether at the temple at Epidaurus or in a moment of immediate crisis on a modern freeway, it is compassion from which the healer moves. Compassion is reinforced through the ritual of claiming a sacred space, and compassion triggers the momentary yet timeless connection of souls. Without it, there is technique or technology—interesting but not healing.

Rollo May

THE EMPATHIC RELATIONSHIP: A FOUNDATION OF HEALING

Rollo May, Ph.D., has for many years been a leader in existential and humanistic psychology. His many popular books include Love and Will *(1969),* Power and Innocence *(1972),* The Courage to Create *(1975),* The Meaning of Anxiety *(1975), and* Freedom and Destiny *(1981). He currently practices in Tiburon, California.*

I n my view, the fundamental element of all healing is empathy. The word *empathy* sounds like *sympathy*, but its meaning is actually quite different. In the present context, it means that the healer does not promote healing in the patient by commiseration or sentimental feeling, but by a kind of subtle communication. In empathy there is a nonverbal interchange of mood, belief, and attitude between doctor and patient, therapist and client, or any two people who have a significant relationship.

Empathy is the experience of understanding that takes place between two human beings. If you go into a music shop and pluck one string of a violin, each of the other instruments in the store will resonate with sound. Similarly, human beings can resonate with each other to such an extent that they can exchange understanding at a subtle level. In extreme terms, this exchange may take the form of telepathy.

Empathy is the basis of both human love and human hatred. It is the way in which one person can intuitively and directly understand or "reach into" another person without using words.

Native peoples in Central Africa serve as a vivid example of the way in which empathy works. In Pygmy societies, when the tribe as a whole believes a person is going to die soon, that person usually does. One explanation is that the force of the tribe's collective mood and attitude exerts a tremendous pressure on the person to die, and he or she usually obliges. Empathy, in this sense, sets the mood for what is going to happen.

Although I have discussed these sorts of destructive effects of empathy in greater detail in *The Meaning of Anxiety* and in *Love and Will,* it is important to mention here that empathy also can produce a positive healing effect. For instance, if a doctor, therapist, or group of individuals believes that a person can be healed, there is a good chance that such healing will occur. As more and more individuals feel that healing is a possibility, the feeling is transferred, through empathy, to the person in need of healing.

The strange thing about healing, however, is that it often occurs with negative emotions as well. Negative emotions can be the trigger for someone to express honest thoughts in psychotherapy and in other healing modalities. In certain cases, negative emotions are essential to the healing process and are the only vehicle capable of taking the patient in a healing direction.

For example, my friend Dr. Irving Yalom, who used to work with people with severe cases of cancer, found that all his patients died except one: a woman who got very angry at her disease. Her anger kept her alive.

Another example of the role of negative emotions in healing can be seen in the work of Alcoholics Anonymous, a group that has taught us much about the effective treatment of alcoholism. One method used by AA is to promote an attitude of despair in the patient. Although we usually regard despair as a negative emotion, it can actually bring a person a sense of humility and a love for a greater power in the universe. We can see, therefore, that emotions we often regard as negative are sometimes the most effective catalysts in particular types of healing.

I have suggested that the empathic relationship is the basis of healing. But because empathy involves the whole spectrum of emotions and attitudes, including negative ones such as anger and despair, it is a mistake to associate healing merely with sympathy. Empathy brings into the healing relationship a range of experience that is far greater than the one to which we are normally accustomed. And the effective therapist must be able to respond to, and bring up to the client, any emotion that is genuinely therapeutic.

Healing should not be oversimplified. It is a complex event filled with great mystery. Effective healers throw themselves into this wondrous and mysterious event with the hope of gaining a greater understanding.

But, although the picture is complex, one can discern predominant themes underlying all healing. Empathy is one of these themes. A healer who is empathic is much more likely to be "present" with a patient and to be genuinely listening to what is occurring at the moment. Such a healer can put aside preconceived notions about what needs to be done, making it easier to discover what the patient really needs. It is with true understanding, gained through empathy, that all effective healing takes place.

Stanley Krippner

TOUCHSTONES OF THE HEALING PROCESS

Stanley Krippner, Ph.D., is professor of psychology and director of the Center for Consciousness Studies at Saybrook Institute in San Francisco. He has authored or coauthored The Realms of Healing, Healing States, Human Possibilities, Dream Telepathy, Song of the Siren, *and* Dreamworking.

M y observations of native healers have taken me to six continents. Over the years I have had the opportunity to witness a great deal of successful healing. I have observed that effective treatment inevitably involves one or more of the following fundamental principles, which make up the common denominators of healing:

1. Certain personal qualities of the practitioner appear to facilitate the client's recovery.
2. Positive client expectations assist healing.
3. A sense of mastery empowers the client.

There is a consensus among healers, therapists, and physicians that some practitioners have personality characteristics that are therapeutic, while others do not. Not only are the actual personal qualities of the practitioner important, but those projected onto him or her by the client are important as well. The process of projection is termed "transference" by psychotherapists and can be a salient factor in the success of therapy.

Carl Rogers observed that while intellectual training and the acquisition of information have many valuable effects on a therapist, they are not correlated with a therapist's success in producing positive outcomes. Rogers found that a therapist's empathy, nonpossessive warmth, and personal genuineness were the factors that most closely related to a client's behavior change.

The second common denominator of healing might be called client expectancy. Abundant evidence from many studies demonstrates its importance. What a person expects to happen in healing often will happen if the expectations are strong enough. In one study, a group of surgical patients were warned before their operations about postoperative pain. They were given breathing exercises to modulate their discomfort. Another group were not given any warnings or exercises. The patients who had been prepared requested only about half as much pain medication as the other group, and left the hospital an average of almost three days sooner.

In 1974, I observed Nemesion Taylo, a Christian spiritualist healer, at work in Manila. His first client that day was an elderly woman, brought in by her grieving relatives, who moaned, "Poor Granny. She's lost her mind. She can't remember our names. She's been possessed by evil spirits." Taylo had her lie down on a table and proceeded to bring his large diamond-chip ring to the tips of her toes and fingers, as well as to her forehead. As Taylo's ring approached her body, the woman would wince with pain. "Yes, it seems to be possession," Taylo muttered, and the relatives nodded in agreement.

For several minutes, Taylo massaged various parts of the old woman's body, moving her limbs upward and downward as he proceeded. He then prayed to Jesus Christ and brought his ring to the client's body parts again. This time she demonstrated no reaction of pain; instead, she smiled at her relatives and, as Taylo pointed to each one, she called out the correct name. As the family joyously left the sanctuary, Taylo whispered to me, "Yes, perhaps the woman was possessed. Or perhaps she just needed a little attention." In this case, the personal qualities of the practitioner served to heighten the positive expectations of the client to produce at least a temporary improvement in her condition.

The final common denominator has to do with a client's sense of mastery, which equips him or her with knowledge about what to do in the future to cope with life's adversities. In physical illness, a patient may feel better and return to work. In addition, the patient may have learned self-regulation, dietary and exercise regimens, and other disease-prevention techniques to avert a recurrence of the ailment. As for psychological problems, the client may have learned the proper prayers that counteract malevolent spirits, the healthy attitudes that counteract depression and anxiety, or the dream interpretation techniques that provide personal empowerment.

Learning and mastery are important components of healing. In addition, they demonstrate the difference between "curing" (removing the symptoms of an ailment and restoring a client to health) and "healing" (attaining wholeness of body, mind, emotions, and spirit). In other words, a patient might be incapable of being cured because his illness is terminal or chronic. Yet that same patient could be healed mentally, emotionally, and spiritually as a result of being taught by the practitioner to review his life, find meaning in it, and become reconciled to death, or by learning how to minimize and manage the distress of a chronic condition.

I first met Rolling Thunder, a medicine man who lives in Nevada, in 1970 and have since observed him conduct several healing sessions and consultations. Once I listened to him give instructions to a client who had come for dream interpretation. Instead of telling the client what the dream meant, Rolling Thunder asked the client to imagine himself as each of the characters in the dream so that he would be able to interpret the dream himself. He gave him tools rather than answers.

My observations of native healers have convinced me that their inner wisdom and lore contain many approaches to the healing arts that deserve attention from both Western practitioners and researchers. I have learned from them that the personal qualities of the practitioner, positive client expectations, and a powerful sense of mastery are three of the most important qualities of healing that have stood the test of time. They are, without question, three touchstones of healing.

Part Five

THE ROLE
OF THE HEALER

*No man can reveal to you aught but that
which already lies half asleep
in the dawning of your knowledge.*

Kahlil Gibran

The authors contributing to this section explore a curious paradox: The role of the healer is *not* to do the healing. Instead, healers empower and enable the individual to achieve healing.

Healers are powerful yet passive guides. They must maintain a strong sense of self, yet not let their own egos get in the way. They serve as a reflective mirror, yet as a role model at the same time.

The role of the healer is to facilitate an individual's own self-healing capacities, self-awareness, self-love, and self-expression. The healer's role is to provide trust, love, and presence for the one being healed, for himself and for the healing process. The healer should be present at the physical, emotional, and spiritual levels, and can embrace global concerns as well.

Emmett E. Miller

TRUST AND HONESTY: FOUNDATIONS OF HEALING

Emmett E. Miller, M.D., is medical director of the Cancer Support and Education Center in Menlo Park, California, and a member of the California Self-Esteem Task Force. In addition to producing nationally distributed audio- and videotapes for self-healing and personal growth, he has authored Self-Imagery: Creating Your Own Good Health *and* Software for the Mind.

T wo crucial requirements of the healing process are trust and honesty. By trust I mean that both the healer and the person to be healed have confidence that there is a power within the body that has the capacity to bring about healing when it is given the opportunity to do so. By honesty I mean the healer's willingness to be faithful and true to the spirit of the patient. In my practice I have seen how both of these qualities must be present for any genuine healing to occur. They are key strands in the golden thread that binds together all methods of healing.

In working with a patient, I find that I must concentrate first of all on discovering what that person can do to let go of nonessentials that may be interfering with the expression of the innate healing power of the body and mind. When this has been accomplished, vital energy is freed that can then be focused toward what is most essential. This process is effectively catalyzed by personal integrity or honesty —a dedication and loyalty to the truth by both therapist and patient.

For example, in my own practice I try not to assume that I know what's going on when a person enters my office. Diagnosing and reviewing the patient's history are often misleading and can be used as crutches to give practitioners a false sense of security. So I often have no formula.

This means that I'm usually hopelessly lost for about the first half of each session. If a person comes to see me with a diagnosis of cancer, for instance, how can I know if his real desire is to heal himself, or if he wants help in facing death? So I try to keep any preconceptions out of the session. Only then can I really hear what patients are trying to tell me.

Here patience is indeed a virtue; I must not try to force this communication. I have to wait until I have received the message from the deepest part of the person—for it is that message to which I must respond as a healer.

What is the deeper message? Perhaps this can best be understood by recalling the Hindu concept of *dharma,* which means one's duty to the deepest part of oneself. When I talk to a patient, I listen and watch very carefully in an attempt to hear this message. Other practitioners who have observed my work are often amazed by the intensity of the focus. I am keenly alert to every flicker or quiver of the eyelids, every tiny change in skin color, every alteration of voice tonality. I allow my senses to become attuned to the process under way in this person. In this way, I can perceive when the patient touches the really important aspect of the illness, that aspect connected with the essential being.

This perception is difficult to describe in words. There is a kind of sparkle when it appears, almost like the flash of light that reveals where a crystal is hidden in a pile of ordinary stones, or that moment when you recognize, in a crowd, the face of a friend you have not seen for a long while. When that happens, I immediately encourage the patient to explore his or her current awareness and to tell me more about it.

For example, the patient may be expressing fear about the possibility of losing her job, or anger at her ex-husband. Then, in the midst of this, she may remark casually, "It's certainly not like a walk on the beach."

Then I encourage her to say more: "A walk on the beach?"

Suddenly, the tears may start to flow, and the patient begins to talk about an experience of contact with nature as a child and about how alive she used to feel.

This is where the challenge of being faithful to the real spirit of the person becomes most important. It is again a matter of honesty, a refusal to settle for less than the whole truth. This means that instead of allowing patients to choke back their tears and forget about the painful thoughts and emotions, I try to create space in which they can share their feelings and explore the sadness in greater depth.

Of course they're sad; they haven't let themselves feel alive for a long time. But until they allow themselves to feel sad, they won't be able to allow themselves to feel alive. Their current mental, physical, emotional, and spiritual problems are connected with resisting that feeling, and with it comes the awareness that can heal.

So healing depends on finding out what is the really living part of the patient, what is most essential, what is closest to the source of that person's spirit. After it is discovered, a personal connection with it is nurtured.

In my own work I find that my own life experiences, if I am willing to be open to them, help me see how to make this connection. Because when I look at that living part of the patient, I usually see some part of myself that I love deeply.

It is often at this point that patients begin to realize there is someone else who cares about them and knows what their problem is like. They perceive that another person has been in the same place, felt the same pain, experienced the same sadness, known the same joy, and they are no longer alone. When empathy or compassionate rapport is allowed to develop in this way, a deep bond is created. It is this bond that is the real basis of effective healing therapy. The work can then proceed freely, and it becomes easier to explore the question of what kinds of thoughts, images, words, deeds, medications, nutrition, or exercises will support this most essential aspect of the person.

The healing process consists of finding, touching, and loving this deepest sense of the patient. It can be summed up in these steps:

(1) Self-awareness. The therapist cannot pretend to know what the patient needs without knowing first who the patient is. For example, in order to recover, does he need to move out of the city or move into the city? Will healing require that she raise a child or decide not to have children? It is crucial to discover the essence of the individual one is treating.

(2) Self-acceptance.   Not long ago a woman came to me who was very angry with herself. She felt that she was no good because, in spite of her best efforts to make her relationships work, they just weren't turning out right. Consequently, she had no sense of her own value. In her own eyes, she was worthless.

I asked her, "If you could have the perfect kind of relationship, what would it look like?" She proceeded to tell me how loving her relationship would be, how it would be based on mutual honesty and respect, how she would instill certain values in her children, and so forth.

I then asked her to suppose that everybody felt that way. If everyone created exactly that kind of relationship and raised their children in that way, would the world be different from the way it is now? She laughed and said that the world would be a wonderful place.

I pointed out to her that what she wanted most, from the deepest part of herself, was something which, if everyone else accepted it, would bring peace, love, and joy to the world. "If that exists in you, at the center," I asked, "how can you tell me you don't have any value?" She got the message, an inner realization took place, and the door to major personal changes was opened.

By helping patients get to know who they really are, what they value and why, we clear the way for self-acceptance, which follows immediately. But people have to be guided to this insight because they have lost track of the deeper parts of themselves. They must first become reacquainted with themselves in order to begin accepting and appreciating themselves. Then self-respect follows almost by definition.

(3) Self-confidence.   A sense of resonance and harmony with one's deepest self arises when the patient sees that the essential part of himself can be trusted. When that occurs, the patient is not far from the final step.

(4) Self-expression.   This step represents the freedom and confidence to express those deepest values of the essential self.

So there is a logical progression that starts with self-awareness and ends with self-expression. But the term self-expression does not refer only to the ability to express oneself in words or even in deeds. Rather, it refers to every kind of activity or behavior, including "internal actions," such as thoughts and emotions, and also to one's physical health, which may be thought of as a kind of behavior (or expression) of the body. When one truly expresses one's essential self, health is a natural by-product.

Healing, in this sense, does not only mean that the physical function returns to normal. Such an arbitrary definition is impossible once we begin thinking in terms of whole persons who are composed of mind, emotion, and spirit as well as body. From this standpoint, health necessarily involves the coordination and congruence of all aspects of one's being, including communications and relationships with others and with the environment. It embraces every aspect of life, including diet, exercise, work, play, and relaxation.

This wholeness, however, depends on an *internal congruence*—an agreement between what we think, feel, and say, so they all fit together without contradiction. This internal harmony, in turn, is only possible when one acts from the deepest part of one's being, from what we are referring to as the essential self. In this way we can see that true health is a natural by-product of honest self-expression or integrity.

When we become healthy in this way, as an outgrowth of self-expression, it becomes possible to live in an ecological balance with our environment. Our sense of wholeness will begin to extend beyond our physical form and embrace the world surrounding us in wider and wider circles of relationships.

As a person gains more strength, he or she naturally starts to include the family and community in that sense of healing and wholeness, until it eventually extends to the totality of mankind, and to all life on the planet.

This continual transcendence of limitations and boundaries is another quality of healing. So when we approach our work as healers (recalling that this is by definition a full-time job) with the qualities of trust and honesty, we will move unerringly toward the source.

A patient or client is, in a way, like a stained-glass window: The presenting symptoms, neuroses, or complaints are like little yellow panes. We must see them but not allow ourselves to be distracted by them, for only by standing back so that we can see the other colors can we truly appreciate the wholeness of the picture.

Ultimately, with perseverance and faith, we may be blessed with a fuller experience and appreciation of the light that, though not directly visible, illuminates the window from the other side. It is the source of this light that is both the means and end of healing.

Dolores Krieger

THE TIMELESS CONCEPT OF HEALING

Dolores Krieger, Ph.D., R.N., a pioneer in therapeutic touch, is a professor at New York University and author of Therapeutic Touch *and* Therapeutic Touch: Healing as a Lifestyle.

T here are endless varieties of healing methods, perhaps as many as the ways in which humans can compassionately relate to one another. In my travels, I have had the good fortune to become close friends with healers from many cultures. In our discussions about the healing process, I have invariably been impressed that we are more alike than different in our experiences with people who are ill, and in our impressions regarding the dynamics of those experiences.

A common recognition among healers is that there are multiple realities, reflecting the multifold states of consciousness at our command. Which reality we relate to depends largely on the predominant facet of consciousness through which we choose to perceive our interactions with the universe. Therefore, each person lives, ultimately, in his or her own reality. Nevertheless, there are common linkages of thought that declare our bonds of human relationship and tie us all together. This is true in all our endeavors, including, especially, the healing act.

Those who have had wide experience in helping or healing people who are ill are often impressed by what we might call ordering principles. These principles are generally little understood but seem to be rooted in the foundations of the healing process. Examples abound. We need only observe the healing of a wound—say, a small but deep cut on the hand—to note with wonder that it often heals without a scar or other indication that anything once marred the intact tissue. Even at this gross level of direct observation, this would seem to be a valid indication of an organizing factor at work.

If we were to examine the healing process at a microscopic level, however, our appreciation would increase considerably. We would realize that the healing process involves several different levels of organization; the materials for seven cellular layers are apparently routed to the correct places as the tissues mend and become fully functional again. As we study this process more deeply, it becomes increasingly clear that certain less obvious, although equally significant, factors are dynamically engaged.

Synchronization is one such factor. In the example of the healing wound, several biochemical substances must be brought into action at the molecular level on a schedule that is exquisitely synchronized. Yet, while we may observe and marvel at the process, it does raise a provocative and profound question: Who—or perhaps what—is the master choreographer of these finely tuned processes that are so closely bound to the healing act?

We see that timing, as well as time, seems to be fundamental to the ordering principles that underlie healing. After twenty years of continued research on healing, and replication of certain experiments by myself and others, I remain awed by repeated demonstrations that time is used differently in the healing act than it appears in linear chronological time.

My own approach to healing, therapeutic touch, remains as it was conceived sixteen years ago, a contemporary interpretation of some ancient healing practices. The major assumptions underlying it are similar to those that provide the foundation for many healing practices. The most basic assumption is that the human being is an open system, a supposition with which life scientists agree.

A second premise is based on a general agreement among non-allopathic healing modalities that illness represents an imbalance in the individual's energy systems. The charge to the healer is to rebalance those systems.

A third proposition says that human beings are capable of both transformation and transcendence, which is essentially the definition of healing.

Over the years, my colleague Dora Kunz and I have found two

characteristics to be consistent in the committed healer: compassion and intentionality. The case for compassion speaks for itself. Intentionality implies that the healer not only exerts his or her will to heal an individual, but also perceives a context in which that healing can take place. This assures that the healing practice will be done in a conscious and conscientious manner.

My view of the direction healing will take in the future comes as a result of a convergence of ideas. My research with families who practice therapeutic touch and my experiences in teaching have led me to the proposition that healing in the future will not only be more concerned with a deeper understanding of the therapeutic functions of the human energy field, but will also tend to occur within a family environment as a social force. Should this occur, I think that the values of compassion and order that are common among those who would be healers will affect society significantly, perhaps in ways not yet dreamed.

The healer recognizes the possibilities for transformation and transcendence of life conditions. He realizes that, as human energy fields, we do not stop at our skin; we flow into one another and, indeed, cannot stand apart. The family would seem an ideal setting for such understanding to grow and flourish as its members care for themselves and one another in empathic, healing ways. From within the family structure and in society at large, such awareness could presage a life-affirmative stance that would be an eloquent statement of compassionate concern of human being for human being and, indeed, for all life.

Elisabeth Kübler-Ross

THE FOUR PILLARS
OF HEALING

Elisabeth Kübler-Ross, M.D., has been at the cutting edge of work in the field of death, dying, and transition for more than twenty years. Her books include On Death and Dying, *an international best-seller, and* AIDS: The Ultimate Challenge. *She is based in Head Waters, Virginia, where she is planning a center for babies with the AIDS virus.*

In my view there are four essential qualities of a healer: trust, faith, love, and humility. The healer must act as a channel—that is, as the conduit of a healing entity or force, whether one calls this God, Christ, the Inner Teacher, or whatever. In order to become such a channel, the healer must have absolute trust in its healing power as well as faith that he or she is capable of channeling it. And, although different healers may channel the healing energy by a variety of different techniques, none of them can heal—no matter what their technique—unless they use it with love and humility.

Love is perhaps the most problematic of these requirements, because all healers have days when they are not open to love. There are no cookbook recipes for staying open to love. What helps one person may not help another.

In my own case, working on my farm and garden, feeding the animals and cultivating the flowers, keeps me grounded and in touch with life, birth, and death, so that after a day or two of farming and gardening I can go back and function as a healer.

Healers must understand that *love* does not only mean love for others; it also means love for oneself. We must be aware of our limits and know when it is necessary to nurture ourselves. Each of us has different ways of nurturing. Some people need people; others need to be alone. We must strike a balance between what we do for ourselves and what we do for others, learning to receive as well as to give. For if we only give and never receive, we get out of balance.

Humility is also very important. Perhaps the greatest need of therapists is to work on eliminating their arrogance. Too often the therapist thinks he or she is the only one who can heal. This is a very divisive attitude. A therapist must have humility enough to know that no one can be a teacher without also being a student; no one can heal without being healed; when we give, we receive; and when we teach, we learn.

With humility a therapist will see that patients know a lot more about themselves than anybody else knows. But if therapists come to a treatment session with the attitude, "I am the therapist, you are the patient," then perhaps 75 percent of their potential effectiveness is already lost. They must be humble enough to know that they, too, need healing. If they are too arrogant to acknowledge this, the whole interaction is contaminated.

The role played by the healer—that is, the type of channeling in which he or she engages—depends on the kind of healing in question. There is a great difference between emotional and physical healing. In my workshops, for instance, I aim at an emotional healing of old, unresolved wounds involving grief, guilt, unfairness, injustice, and so forth. In this kind of healing, my role is to be a catalyst. I simply am there to help people get in touch with the "unfinished business" of their old wounds and pain, and to push them into it as deeply as they can go so they can get it out of their systems by externalizing it.

For every kind of unfinished business there is a particular form of externalization that is most appropriate. With fear, for example, screaming is most effective; with hatred and repressed anger, it can help to beat up a phone book and shred it to pieces. With grief, I encourage people to cry and wail. With guilt, they share their feelings with a group of nonjudgmental people who practice (but don't preach) unconditional love. If guilt is shared, and if it is genuine, then this is followed by a flood of tears that washes the guilt away and leaves a feeling of forgiveness.

All of these methods are in the realm of emotional healing. In emotional healing the therapist needs to use all the expertise and techniques in which he has been trained, such as those just described.

But I do not know exactly how physical healing occurs, because it happens spontaneously and at the least expected moments.

For example, at one of my workshops a huge man, weighing perhaps four hundred pounds, suddenly and unexpectedly went into an acute homicidal rage. I could see that I had to rescue a woman who was much too close to him. I stepped forward and pushed her away, but in the process the man brought a rubber hose (which was supposed to be used to take out anger on a phone book) down on my bare toes with all his strength, crushing them.

I could not stop to focus on the pain. I capped my big toe with my hand, ignoring the pain, and focused all my energy on the enraged man in order to push him even further into the depths of his rage, so he could go all the way through it and get it out. Then, suddenly, he was over it and the group was safe.

I found myself wondering why I was sitting in such a strange position, pulling my right knee up and holding my big toe. Remembering what had happened, I took my hand away to look at my toe, expecting the worst. To my amazement, there was no trace of any injury. It had been instantaneously healed.

I have had several other experiences of spontaneous physical healing in emergency situations. In each case, the reason I was able to heal myself was that I did not have time to think. As a physician I have been trained to believe that such instantaneous healing cannot happen. But in emergencies, when we have to focus totally on the situation and have no time to think, we do not block our innate potential for self-healing—a potential that I believe each of us has. If we would develop more trust and faith in our own inner healing ability, spontaneous physical healing could occur more often.

Healing does not necessarily mean to become physically well or to be able to get up and walk around again. Rather, it means achieving a balance between the physical, emotional, intellectual, and spiritual dimensions. For example, five-year-old children who have been sick with leukemia for two or three years are often very spiritually awake. It seems that the longer they suffer physically, the more the spiritual dimension opens up and the more intuitive they become. They give the impression of a very old, wise soul who has much more knowledge of life than, say, a fifty- or sixty-year-old. At the end of their lives, these children with leukemia have little or no pain. They are emotionally sound, and on an intellectual level they can share things it is almost impossible to believe could come from a child. To me this is a healing, although they are not well from our earthly point of view.

Many AIDS patients, even more so than patients suffering from cancer or other life-threatening illnesses, are lacking in qualities of self-worth, self-esteem, and self-trust. These are blocked by a lot of guilt, shame, and ambivalence. Therefore, we first help them to get rid of their negativity, using the same techniques used in other workshops but at a much more intense level. Then, once they learn to love themselves and trust themselves, the spiritual dimension begins to open up. Only then are they ready for healing.

Healing does not occur only at an individual level. Because each individual is connected through a vast network of relationships to innumerable other people and creatures on the planet, the process of healing even one person has far-reaching ramifications.

It seems to me that the whole planet is a terminally ill patient at this time. Most people know that global levels of stress are building to a dangerous point, and the planet is threatened by nuclear destruction and environmental catastrophe. The conclusion is that there must inevitably be a global cleansing to eliminate the hatred, greed, pain, grief, and rage that have been repressed for so long. In other words, a process similar to the one that occurs in my workshops must happen to the planet as a whole if the earth is to survive.

Don Hanlon Johnson

PRESENCE

Don Hanlon Johnson, Ph.D., is director of the graduate studies program in somatic psychology and education at Antioch University and coordinator of the somatics program at Esalen Institute. He is the author of Body *and* The Protean Body *and serves as a contributing editor of the journal* Somatics.

When I think of the golden thread that unites healers, I recall the *presence* of the late psychologist Carl Rogers, his eyes really seeing me, his ears fully taking in my words; of Ida Rolf, the founder of Rolfing, present in her fingers to the most subtle message of my muscles; of psychiatrist Milton Erickson, slumped catlike in his wheelchair, alert to the least gesture or shift of eye; of the Tibetan Buddhist teacher Trungpa Rimpoche, even when tipsy on sake still fully conscious in his cosmic humor.

I spent some fourteen years of my life as a Jesuit seminarian and priest, in large part because the first time I encountered true presence was with a Jesuit priest. After twenty-one years of being around people who seemed to be "somewhere else," meeting someone who was just "here" was so illuminating that I hungered for what he had found.

This encounter contained the seeds of what I was later to understand about the healing power of simple presence. Our discontents grow within a world of family, church, school, and business, where we experience only the flimsiest contact with each other. We are usually so occupied with our own business, chattering to ourselves, immured in our own pain and worries, that we are incapable of simply being there with each other for more than a brief moment. And even when we are, we find it almost impossible to let others know, to express our felt contact with them.

"Expression" means pressing out what is inside, moving it outside of myself so that I begin to contact others. Only when I press my inner world out to the surfaces of my eyes, ears, and hands, can I come into true contact with you.

The dazzling successes of the great teachers and therapists and the unfamiliar quality of their presence have led to a mistaken belief that their success lies in their techniques. Obsession with technique divides healers into sects and obscures the nature of what heals. For example, Moshe Feldenkrais who created a type of bodywork called Feldenkrais Technique, taught that learning about others by watching them, moving their limbs, paying close attention to what they actually do, is the essence of therapy. But instead of teaching his students how to pay attention in a nonjudgmental way, he taught hundreds of specific exercises and even added to their arsenal of judgments. Although Zen teacher Suzuki Roshi taught that the path to reality is methodless, his students are often obsessed with forcing their bodies into preconceived postures.

Two pure forms of teaching presence applied to therapy and education can be found in the work of Carl Rogers and Charlotte Selver. Both have taught that the only goal of the therapist is *being there for what is.* Difficulties in transmitting their genius reveal how hard it is to comprehend presence. To be truly present with another person, I must find what interests me, what distracts me from my busy inner world, which is flooded with chatter and images. Rogers was fascinated by listening; I am not, feeling restless after a short while of listening to someone talk. Selver is endlessly fascinated by students' bare perceptions—of what it is like to lift a foot, or to glide the palm of a hand along a patch of grass. Those things fascinate me, too, but few people seem to share that fascination. Most find such fragile sensations boring and insignificant.

The path to presence is through what grabs our attention about other people and the outside world. For one person, it may be imagery; for another, the intricacies of verbal language, or nonverbal expression, skin texture, or styles of movement.

Once we have learned to follow that fascination, we can benefit by expanding our field of interest to include other aspects of reality. In fact, failure to expand the scope of presence often severely limits a particular therapy. Carl Jung could not take the body seriously, leaving a group of followers who are only today beginning to recover it at the most rudimentary level. Sigmund Freud and Wilhelm Reich could not be present to a person's spiritual aspirations. Ida Rolf became impatient when her manipulations of fascia plunged a person into strong emotions. Fritz Perls, a founder of Gestalt therapy, was so absent from a person's philosophical or political passions that he even became contemptuous of them.

The great mistake—one that infects world politics as well as the family of therapies—has been when we take what is fascinating to us, the aspects of reality to which we are present, as the real, normative, or ideal, and dismiss other dimensions as illusion.

Presence, in fact, is a useful principle for appreciating the contributions of a particular method to the whole, and for building a more adequate theory for the education of therapists. Freud's analysis of transference and countertransference and Reich's theory of character armor provide major strategies for loosening the veils created by personal history, which keep us from being in contact with what is. Jung's archetypal psychology can enable us to dip into the profound currents of energy that sweep us out of the private into contact with the collective. F. M. Alexander, Moshe Feldenkrais, and Ida Rolf teach us how to move out of the rigid patterns that separate us from each other into the supple movements necessary for intimate contact. Feminist therapists such as Nancy Chodorow and Jean Baker Miller show how gender roles create a world dangerously polarized between isolation and symbiosis, with neither men nor women knowing the alternative of presence to each other as equals.

The notion of presence links contemporary Western therapies to more ancient approaches of human development. The psychophysical techniques of Asia, the Middle East, and European monasticism (such as meditation practices, chants, and movement rituals) are aimed at the state of mindfulness, in which the student learns to be present to what is.

But the history of those spiritual traditions has some important lessons about the traps on the way to presence. In every tradition, men and women experimenting with methods of contacting what is have repeatedly ended up encapsulated within formal systems. Instead of passing on their excitement about discovering what's real, they created communities dedicated to security at the price of truth.

The challenge that faces us is whether we can profit from what the founders of Judaism, Christianity, Hinduism, Buddhism, Islam, and shamanism did not have—a sense of history, anthropology, science, gender and ethnic issues, economics, and democratic process—

in order to engage in a more collaborative shaping of the world, instead of making further contributions to the sectarianism that threatens our survival. Presence entails fully knowing that babies, women, and the old are starving and being maimed by militarism justified by high ideals; that forests and seas are dying; that there are fewer butterflies in our gardens, and more homeless on our streets.

Michael Harner

THE HIDDEN UNIVERSE OF THE HEALER

Michael Harner, Ph.D., is head of the Foundation for Shamanic Studies in Norwalk, Connecticut. He is a professor and former chairman of the Anthropology Department of the Graduate Faculty at the New School for Social Research in New York. His books include The Way of the Shaman, The Jivaro, *and* Hallucinogens and Shamanism.

I n my practice of shamanism I have learned that shamanic healing depends on communicating in a humble and heartfelt way with the awesome power of the universe. Although spiritual healers in different times and cultures may use many superficially different techniques, I believe each of them must somehow gain access to a hidden reality to transmit the power and wisdom of the universe to others who are in need.

Successful healers everywhere work in ways that are right for them and the people they help. After all, as human beings we understand the hidden reality in ways that reflect our own personal and group histories. For example, I know a famous healer in India who works by making a conscious link with a certain Hindu saint. For her, this is the right method of establishing communication with the underlying power of the universe because, as a Hindu, her concentration on this saint brings a feeling and awareness to her heart that gives her access to the greater power of the universe. But for a shaman in a tribal culture, a different kind of spiritual linkage analogous to that saint may be required. It may involve a sacred plant, or even a rock, such as a quartz crystal. Whatever its form, it will be something that is deeply heartfelt and honored by the healer.

Such a link opens the heart of the healer to such a degree that he or she "disappears," in a sense, from the scene. That is, the link allows the healer to substantially lose his or her ego, and therefore the healer feels no need to take credit for the healing. The link, in a sense, substitutes for the healer's ego. Achieving such an attitude is crucial, because to the degree that a healer remains in ordinary, ego-oriented reality, he or she is interfering with the miracle-producing power inherent in the universe.

My views on this subject have been molded by many miraculous experiences over the years. As these experiences accumulate, more pieces fit together and gradually become less and less puzzling— although, of course, there is always the ultimate Mystery.

One of the distinctive healing methods of the shaman involves entering an altered state of consciousness to make what is known as a "journey" into the hidden dimension of the universe, or nonordinary reality. In nonordinary reality shamans may journey to the Lower World or the Upper World, regions they believe we go to at death and from which we emerge at birth. In other words, shamans are able to travel beyond the limits that define reality for most people.

In these journeys, the shaman seeks communication and aid from spirit representatives. Through contact with them, the shaman can bring back knowledge for the benefit of others in his community (for example, knowledge of how to diagnose and heal a particular illness), as well as powerful inner knowledge.

In his classic book *Shamanism: Archaic Techniques of Ecstasy,* Mircea Eliade points out that the shamanic journey is one of the most characteristic spiritual aspects of shamanism. It can be facilitated by a variety of tools and techniques. These often involve the use of monotonous percussion sounds, such as drumming, which has the power of altering one's state of consciousness and allowing access to this other, hidden reality.

From a shamanic point of view, so-called ordinary reality is a reality of conflict, pain, and suffering. There can be peak experiences in this reality, but they are not the most predominant feature. In nonordinary reality, however, the most prevalent aspect is ecstatic experience. As the shaman journeys farther and farther, he or she approaches the ineffable experience of shamanic ecstasy, moving beyond the realm of time, and becoming aware of a fundamental egolessness, finally merging and becoming one with the universe itself.

Between the extremes of nonordinary and ordinary reality, the shaman works with "intermediaries" or "representatives" in the spiritual realm, moving back and forth between the two realities in order to help people experience the deeper harmony within themselves, to heal pain and disharmony.

A related distinctive feature of shamanism, as compared with certain contemporary self-help methods of healing, is that the shaman intercedes for someone other than himself. This concept of compassionate intervention is a key feature of shamanism and is found at all levels of practice. Even the most advanced shamans typically have other shamans who work on their behalf when they need help.

Working in harmony in an egoless way will bring the best results. This is a major reason why shamans emphasize helping and being helped by others, working in harmony together as a community. They typically work in a healing circle, sitting together, focusing their energy to help others, playing the drum, with the shaman and the patient in the center of the circle. The circle also symbolizes the underlying harmony and connectedness of all things.

Healing, however, is not only one-way. In the process of serving the community, the shaman is also helped with his own problems. Many times, while working to help others, the members of a circle will find themselves spontaneously healed of their own pain and illness without even asking for help.

The shaman typically has more immediate knowledge of the healing power of the universe than other members of the community, having become familiar with it by making "journeys." The shaman can perceive what others cannot and can converse with entities hidden from others. The shaman has the conscious, firsthand connection that makes him a valuable human resource in the community.

Tribal shamans were the specialists who ventured into the hidden dimension. But other spiritual specialists were involved in the healing process as well: Older people in the tribe were often skilled with pharmaceuticals such as plant remedies; others were skilled at bone-setting, others at massage, and still others were masters of ritual. In other words, the ancient approach to healing was usually complementary and holistic.

Today we are starting to see a movement back to a more holistic approach. The rising interest of Europeans and Americans in shamanism points to the fact that in our research for a holistic approach, we are rediscovering value in the classic shamanic practices of visualization and altering states of consciousness. We are beginning to recognize that our ancestors had developed valuable systems. As this recognition develops, I believe there will be greater movement toward supplementing orthodox medicine with time-tested methods of spiritual healing such as shamanism.

Janet F. Quinn

HEALING: THE EMERGENCE OF RIGHT RELATIONSHIP

Janet F. Quinn, Ph.D., R.N., is an associate professor of nursing at the University of South Carolina. She has been involved in the practice, teaching, and research of therapeutic touch since 1976. She has authored numerous articles and book chapters on therapeutic touch and has conducted workshops throughout the United States and Canada.

The root of the word *heal* is the Anglo-Saxon word *haelen,* which means to be or to become whole. It is clear that wholeness as it relates to human beings is much too encompassing to be constrained by or in the physical world. So the absence of any physical parts or the loss of function of any of those parts does not negate wholeness, just as the presence and proper functioning of these same parts does not ensure wholeness.

Popular wisdom tells us that healing and health concern "harmony of body-mind-spirit." If we can move beyond the jargon and begin to apprehend the deeper sense of those words, we can move closer to understanding wholeness, at least intuitively.

The word *harmony* can be found in a thesaurus as a synonym for *connection.* Other synonyms for connection are relationship, congruity, and unification; synonyms for harmony include unity, order, peace, and reconciliation. If we consider and reconsider these words, allowing them to gently wash over us and settle into our consciousness, they begin to weave themselves into a rich and meaningful tapestry. The image that emerges suggests that when we talk about wholeness, we are talking fundamentally about relationship.

This relatedness is the opposite of alienation, isolation, estrangement, and fragmentation. Any or all of these can occur at different levels of human existence, with or without our conscious awareness. We can be alienated from our bodies, from our own deepest self, from our closest friends, or from society. No matter at what level, when we are alienated or isolated, we are not whole; we are dis-eased. When true healing occurs, relationship is reestablished.

Given this conceptualization of healing, what facilitates the process? Are there universal principles of healing?

Most important, we can observe that the locus of healing is within the patient. Healing, no matter what the intervention, is not something that can be given or owned by the practitioner or therapist. All healing, without exception, is self-healing.

We labor under the myth that it is the ministrations of health-care providers that cure or heal people. This is simply an illusion, a product of faulty logic. The assumption is that if a patient gets well *after* surgery, she gets well *because* of surgery. The reality is that surgery does not cure/heal. Drugs do not cure/heal. Acupuncture, or crystals, or homeopathy do not cure/heal. The person who undergoes the surgery, or takes the drug, or receives the alternative treatment must heal herself. Any or all of the above-named ministrations may be necessary to remove barriers to self-healing or to stimulate it, but they are not sufficient causes for healing. We know clinically and anecdotally that this is true. We know of patients who die despite "successful" surgery.

Healing is a total, organismic, synergistic response that must emerge from within the individual if recovery and growth are to be accomplished. I have coined the term the Haelen Effect to refer to the totality of the healing response. The Haelen Effect is characterized by, among other things, the system's principle of equifinality: Many pathways can lead to the same end point. The Haelen Effect can be stimulated by a host of different external interventions or by none at all. The elicitation of the effect, the total organismic response toward wholeness, is the goal of any healing intervention.

Intervention designed to accomplish this goal begins with the least invasive approaches available and only then, if necessary, progresses to more invasive measures. Because the locus of healing lies within the individual, the distinction between "real" and "placebo" treatments or effects is a false one. All treatments are stimuli for the

Haelen Effect, and any one may be more or less effective for any given person. Surgery and drugs are not the only forms of "real" treatment. Alternative healing interventions cannot be dismissed as trivial or capable of producing only "placebo" effects.

In addition to changing the way we think about interventions, this concept of the locus of healing causes a fundamental shift in thinking about the role of the therapist. Within this concept of healing, the therapist functions in the capacity of what can best be described as a midwife. (I would ask the reader to ignore here the gender associated with the term and simply consider the role, which is filled by both men and women.) The midwife is one who assists in the birthing process, bringing forth new life, new relationship. This is what is inherently involved in the healing interaction.

When true healing occurs, there is always new life arising. Healing is creative, bringing forth patterns and connections that did not exist before. Rather than a simple returning to some prior level of being, healing involves emergence, and during emergence a midwife is needed, not a surgeon. Rather than imposing onto the system, a midwife allows the system to move in its own ways; she doesn't force, but facilitates; doesn't push, but receives; doesn't insist, but accepts. The midwife is prepared to take more active steps, but only when they become essential.

The midwife embraces emergence with a fundamental trust in the wisdom of the process and of the body. She represents a safe place into which the new life may emerge. She holds new life with awe and reverence, and claims no credit for its miraculous arrival, satisfied to have been present for the journey.

Contrast the images that arise in your mind reading the above description with those created by the following: "We're going to fight this thing; we're going to win the war on cancer; this is the strongest drug you can get." It should be clear that we are dealing with two very different states of mind that demand two different roles for the therapist. One is designed to cure disease; one is about birthing health/wholeness.

No suggestion is made here that we discard conventional treatment of disease. Rather, I am suggesting that we need to be conscious of these distinctions and, when we seek healing, to respond with approaches that are appropriate for eliciting the Haelen Effect.

Today our diseases are increasingly those of the spirit, yet our treatments are more and more biophysical. Our sick-care institutions now advertise to convince us that they can provide the "best care possible." This means that the institutions have what they consider the biggest or the newest machines with which to attack disease. Care has become synonymous with the provision of things and procedures, in spite of the fact that 80 percent of the problems people present for medical treatment are self-limiting, and thousands of people visit physicians' offices every year just to be touched.

Nurses, who traditionally have provided human-to-human caring, are leaving the health-care system in droves. Why? Because they entered it to be healers, midwives to the healing process, but they have found themselves taking care of machines instead.

I believe that these circumstances are the consequence of a culture in which the feminine principle has been ignored and devalued. We are sadly out of balance and out of right relationship. The feminine principle is deeply concerned with nurturing relationship. Nurses' work has traditionally been women's work and has not been highly valued by society. Yet healing work always represents the feminine in action, regardless of the gender of the healer.

It is abundantly clear that if we continue on our course of increasing isolation and alienation, we will self-destruct. The system fosters this attitude by maintaining absolute authority in matters of health and illness. However, that system can no longer afford such a posture economically, socially, or ethically. It must begin to release its grip.

Healing in the future must involve major shifts in the way we think about health and illness. The focus of a health-care system must be on facilitating wholeness, which means facilitating right relationship. The techniques are beside the point. What must occur is twofold: the revaluing of the feminine principle and its ways, and the empowerment of individuals and communities to create their own health and healing.

The most important role that health-care practitioners will fill in the future will be an educational one. At the very least, communities must be given the opportunity to learn how to become their own healers. For example, we need community healing centers staffed by volunteer senior citizens who have been taught therapeutic touch or the use of imagery or massage. We could decrease the costs of health care dramatically by teaching people how to heal each other.

This is only one aspect of the effects of such a plan. We need only imagine the type of community bonding that might develop in such circumstances, and consider the consequences for planetary healing. As one enters into the process of becoming a healer, one is changed irrevocably. As the feminine is allowed to emerge, one begins to appreciate the miracle and sacredness of life and the fundamental unity among people. This awareness of the whole, this right relationship with ourselves and with our environment, is the only hope we have for planetary survival. Relationship is not just pleasant or something to "get" after we've earned enough money or prestige. We will either be healed, emerging into right relationship with ourselves and our planet, or we will die.

When we consider directions for healing in the future, we can no longer ask, "What can healers do to serve humanity?" We must ask, "How can we turn all of humanity into healers?" I would suggest that there is only one answer. We must become focused in our commitment to empowerment, and in so doing we must acknowledge, revere, and allow the reemergence and revaluing of the feminine. We have no choice, and the time is short.

Part Six

THE HEALING ATTITUDE

We are what we think.
All that we are arises with our thoughts.
With our thoughts we make the world.
The Buddha

A positive, life-affirming attitude is a key in the healing process. Each contributor in this section describes the role that overcoming negative mental obstacles plays in a person's ability to be healed.

Reading the following pieces, you will sense that a changed attitude can be the greatest healing that can take place. In other words, effective healing stems as much from a changed perception as from a changed body. A complete and true healing comes from within the person in need. If a person is healed from within, the body may or may not change. At some level, it may not matter, for the real work has begun.

A healing attitude is not superficial. It involves a deep inner knowledge that we are not victims of the world. Rather, we have the authority to respond to adversity in any way we choose. By taking responsibility for our health and for our entire lives, we gain a sense of mastery over what we previously perceived as beyond our control. These contributors show us how emotions such as anger, greed, and fear need to be replaced with personal responsibility, acceptance, selflessness, and love.

Sun Bear

HEALING ATTITUDES

Sun Bear is medicine chief of the Bear Tribe Medicine Society based in Spokane, Washington, which he founded in 1970. He is the author of Sun Bear: The Path of Power *(with Wabun)*, At Home in the Wilderness, The Medicine Wheel: Earth Astrology *(with Wabun and Nimishosha), and* Buffalo Hearts.

I want to discuss two of the most important factors involved in healing: overcoming negative blocks, and developing positive, life-affirming attitudes. Perhaps the best way to approach these ideas is to show how they are involved in my own practice.

When someone comes to me for healing or help, the first thing I do is to examine the overall pattern of the person's life. This usually reveals certain blocks that are holding him or her back from being healed. These blocks may be present on both a physical and a spiritual level.

From the spiritual standpoint, the most common blocks are the negative attitudes and emotions that a lot of people carry around all the time. These blocks must be overcome for healing to occur. In working with people who have cancer or other serious illnesses, I find that unless they can learn to let go of negativity, their sickness comes back.

In order to become totally healed, a person has to throw out hatred, envy, jealousy, and other destructive attitudes and feelings. Although such factors start within the mind, they quickly manifest in the body, becoming a stiff shoulder, a sluggish liver, cancer, or other illnesses. I believe that all genuine healing addresses the problem of unblocking negativities in one way or another.

One method I have used successfully to do this is to have people go outdoors, find a place in the earth, and dig a hole. Then they speak into this hole all the things that are bothering them in their lives. If they feel uptight about something concerning their mate or someone else, if they have had rage bottled up for a long time, if they have unexpressed grief or dread, all of this gets dumped into that hole. Thus they give their negativity to the earth.

After the negative attitudes and emotions have been eliminated, they have to be replaced by positive ones. If a healer can create in a person a sense of well-being, a sense that "Life is good for me after all," that person will be on the road to recovery.

Of course, it is very important that the patient should want to get well. A strong desire to heal is a crucial factor in the healing process. One of the best reasons for wanting to get well is the wish to continue enjoying life. So, if people can be brought to feel that they have a right to be happy, that they *deserve* to be happy, and that they are, in fact, already enjoying a happy life, this is one of the most powerful motivators for healing.

This accounts for the fact, which I have observed over many years, that happy people do not get sick as often as sad ones. In fact, people who become depressed and discouraged by the problems of life are already half-sick just by their attitudes. When the healer can break people free of such thought patterns and get them to start enjoying life again, a major step has been taken toward health.

This means that the healer must, in a sense, be a role model for those he or she is trying to help. A sad, negative, or despairing healer is, in my view, a contradiction in terms. I tell people that I personally stay happy at least 97 percent of the time. And I feel that this is indeed my path. Staying happy is a very important part of it. I believe this is why people often say to me, "When you are around, we feel that we are more alive." Being able to communicate and inspire this sense of well-being in others is an important aspect of the healer's art.

The development of positive attitudes in the patient can also be facilitated in a supportive group atmosphere. A suffering person is encouraged and strengthened by the awareness that other people, with serious problems of their own, still care enough to give support. This is especially beneficial in the case of mental or emotional problems. Moreover, a supportive group also can counteract the negative attitudes that may have been instilled in the past by nonsupportive groups.

Unfortunately, it is too often the case in our society that a person gets picked on for having a problem—first by family members, then by acquaintances. The troubled person is like a chicken with a small red speck on its body, which the other chickens peck at until they have seriously injured the chicken. Thus a child may go to school with some minor problem or "difference"—perhaps unusual shyness or a speech difficulty—and the other children pick on him until his problem grows to be a big one. Being in a supportive group is often the best way to heal the scars caused long ago by such experiences.

It is also important that people who wish to be healed should believe the healer has the power to heal them. If the patient believes this, the healer is already halfway home. That is why in my work I am very much concerned with people's belief systems. For instance, some people in Western society may find it difficult to have confidence in a spiritual medicine man who prays over them and performs a ceremony using an eagle feather. Some people may be conditioned to the point where they feel they must have a doctor with an M.D. to prescribe treatment for them. This conditioning may be so strong that it will prevent them from believing that they can be healed in any other way. Getting past such an obstacle can be very difficult.

Usually, however, when I do a healing ceremony for a person and pray over him or her, the Spirit will tell me something that I should do for that person. Sometimes I can sense the person's illness in my own body, at least to some degree, and from this I know what the Spirit wants me to do.

When I work, I channel energy that travels through me from other sources and gets translated as information for the person who is to be healed. I believe there are energies or intelligences in the universe that help the healer. You can call this God, the Great Spirit, Spirit Helpers, or whatever. When I pray I ask for the help of one of those powers. I do not question the messages I receive, and I am not dogmatic about what method must be used. If a particular way works for a patient, that is what I am really interested in.

Thus the openness of the healer is another key element in the therapeutic process. In my own work, for instance, I have never allowed myself to think that I have all the answers. I stress with all my apprentices that they should not get locked into a dogmatic idea or system of any kind. If a healer knows something well and finds that it works, then it is appropriate. It may be a certain ceremony or way

of praying; it may be a particular conceptual system or way of thinking; or it may be a system of dealing with problems, such as Rolfing
or Reichian therapy. Whatever the method, if it works, then it is good.
But this does not mean that one cannot change methods later. In fact,
I know a number of therapists who started out practicing one way
sincerely for a number of years and then moved on to something else
they found to work better. A healer needs to remain open and sensitive to what may be required from moment to moment.

I find in my own work, too, that it is often more effective to
approach a person with an arm over the shoulder rather than with the
confrontational, "get-tough" style advocated in some methods of
therapy. For instance, I have had young men come for healing who
were loud and arrogant. Usually they wonder why other people don't
like them. I sit down with them for a while and explain why they are
having trouble getting along with other people. I present this in a
quiet, nonconfrontational manner—not as a challenge—and this usually works quite well.

When someone comes to me for healing, I also try not to make
him or her feel guilty about the sickness. There is still an unfortunate
tendency in some parts of society for people to think that sickness
means one has done something bad or evil. But one of the common
things shared by all true healers is the attitude that the therapist's job
is simply to help those who come for healing—not to judge, condemn,
or sentence them. This attitude is especially important now, when
illnesses such as AIDS are popular targets for those who would like
to instill guilt or condemnation. The role of the therapist, if nothing
else, is to give the patient some energy and support.

So the attitude of the healer, as well as of the person to be healed,
plays a crucial role in the healing process. This means, of course, that
the healer must enjoy what he or she is doing. In my own case, I enjoy
everything I do, whether it's performing a healing ceremony, giving
a lecture, chopping wood, or cleaning out the chicken barn. The key
here is to be able to live fully in the present moment. Many people
are constantly brooding, wishing they were someplace else, doing
something else—with the result that they are never happy. Such a
person does not make a good healer.

Indeed, no one should be in the healing profession who does not
enjoy it. In working with physicians, psychiatrists, and other therapists, I tell them they need to take off a certain amount of time for
themselves; they must avoid burnout if they are to continue to be
good at what they do. The avoidance of burnout is perhaps more
crucial in healing than in any other profession. This is why I even

suggest to therapists that they have an alternative career, something that gives them a break from the stress of dealing with life-and-death matters.

In the future, I think therapists should become much more conscious of helping people change their lifestyles and habits in such a way that they don't get sick in the first place. I am not overwhelmingly impressed with technological "miracles" like artificial hearts. If scientists can figure out how to keep people from getting heart attacks in the first place, this will be a real achievement. And the first step will be to show people how to move beyond negative conditioning, how to become happy, and how to develop a sense of enjoyment in life.

Gerald Jampolsky

LIVING AND LOVING ONE SECOND AT A TIME

Gerald Jampolsky, M.D., is a psychiatrist and founder of the Center for Attitudinal Healing in Tiburon, California. He has published extensively, including the best-selling books Love Is Letting Go of Fear, Good Bye to Guilt, Teach Only Love, *and* To Give Is to Receive: 18-Day Mini-Course on Healing Relationships.

For me, the common denominator in all healing is God. And because God and love are one and the same, the common denominator in healing is love. To heal and to be healed is to walk each day, each hour, each second with God. It is to recognize that God is our only true relationship. To heal is to recognize every encounter with another person as a holy encounter, seeing only the holiness in that person.

For me, the healing process is made up of unconditional love, forgiveness, and letting go of fear. It is that simple.

I love this quote from *A Course in Miracles:* "Simplicity is very difficult for a twisted mind to understand." I can attest to how confused and twisted my mind can be on this adventure called life.

At the Center for Attitudinal Healing in Tiburon, California, which I helped to create in 1975, we define health and healing quite differently from the conventional health model, which is concerned about the state of the body and its symptoms and has as its goal the healing of the body. At this center and our other forty-five centers worldwide, peace of mind, peace of God, is our only goal. We define health as inner peace, and healing as letting go of fear.

We do our best to create an unconditional loving environment in which everyone is an equal teacher and student to each other. We believe healing is simply seeing no value in negative thoughts such as guilt, fear, anxiety, and worry. We have no gurus. We are there to be witnesses to each other that peace of mind occurs the second we are willing to put all of our energy into helping and giving unconditional love to another. We see both children and adults who have catastrophic illnesses, including AIDS. We also have a large person-to-person program that focuses on healing relationships through forgiveness and not making judgments.

We strive to see only two emotions: love and fear. We choose to retrain our minds not to see the world or those in it as attacking; we choose to see others as either loving or fearful. When they are fearful, they are giving us a call of help for love. We can be loving and compassionate to someone whom we perceive as fearful. But if we choose to see another person as "attacking," we will attack back and in that process attack ourselves. In our healing process, we choose not to see ourselves as victims, and to take responsibility for our thoughts and feelings. In that process, we learn that there is no one to blame.

Most of my life I have been caught in the world's thought system where I was focused on "me" and what I could get, making judgments on people I thought were my friends or enemies. I had outer success but inner chaos and spent an enormous amount of time being fearful of the past and future. I was more focused on achievement and performance than on love.

In 1975, after years of being a militant atheist, I began to experience the presence of God and recognize that my own healing had to do with awakening to the presence of the peace of God and forgiveness. It was then that I was introduced to *A Course in Miracles*, a book that helps on one's pathway of spiritual transformation.

As I look back on my life, no one ever told me or demonstrated for me as a child that if I wanted to have consistent peace of mind, all I had to do was make peace of mind top priority and my only goal. No one ever told me all I had to do is to live one second at a time, being kind, gentle, tender, and loving to all that is living—the human species, animals, insects, plants, trees—and to exclude no one from my love, including myself. It is myself that I am most tempted to leave out, and that is when I become an unhealed healer.

No one ever told me that it was possible to live life in slow motion, one second at a time, as if that second were the only time there was, an eternal second. Or that it would be possible to live that second with the fire of compassion in my heart for living completely devoid of blaming another person or myself and not holding onto guilt or grievances.

Slowly but surely, I am finding that nothing can hurt me except my own thoughts, my own mind. I still feel I am in kindergarten on my spiritual pathway. There is not a day when I don't fall down. But now I find that I can pick myself up and choose love once again, instead of being attached to guilt, anger, depression, and illness. I do my best each day to have peace of God as my only goal and forgiveness as my only function, and to listen to the voice of love, the voice of God within my heart, to tell me what to think, say, and do.

To me, healing is releasing from the past. It is retraining my mind so as not to see the shadow of the past on anyone. It is learning not to make interpretations of people's behavior or motives. It is letting go of the desire to want to change another person. It is letting go of expectations, assumptions, and the desire to control or manipulate another person.

To me, healing is letting God write the script of my life. It is choosing to let God's will and my will be one. This continues to be a struggle for me the moment that I think I know what is best for myself or another person.

Healing is knowing that forgiveness is the key to happiness and offers me everything that I want. Healing is knowing that the only reality in the universe is love, and that love is the most important healer known to the world.

To heal is to trust in a creative force that is loving and forgiving, and to know in our hearts that there is no separation and we are all joined in love with God and each other. It means that all hearts and minds are joined as one.

Healing is letting go of our fear of the concept of death, and recognizing that our true reality is a spiritual one—with no limitations. Healing means letting go of the concept that our identity is limited to a personality and a body that is doomed sooner or later to be hurt, be rejected, get sick, and die.

Healing is to know that life is eternal. There is no death here; it is to awaken ourselves to love and caring for each other.

Healing is letting go of the fearful child so many of us carry inside, and awakening to the innocent child who has always been within us.

To heal is to become a messenger of God, accepting God's love for ourselves and giving that unconditional love to all, with no exceptions.

To heal is to live one's life as a prayer, accepting our natural state of pure joy and happiness, peace and love, and extending that to all life.

For me, the healing process starts at the beginning of the day when I devote twenty minutes to silencing my mind and reminding myself what kind of day I wish to experience—a day devoted to God. I start the day with three passages from *A Course in Miracles*. I would like to share them with you:

> I am not a body. I am free.
> For I am still as God created me.

> The peace of God is my one goal; the aim
> Of all my living here, the end I seek,
> My purpose and my function and my life,
> While I abide when I am not at home.

> I am here only to be truly helpful.
> I am here to represent Him Who sent me.
> I do not have to worry about what to say, or what to
>   do, because He Who sent me will direct me.
> I am content to be wherever He wishes, knowing He
>   goes there with me.
> I will be healed as I let Him teach me to heal.

Another part of my healing process takes place at the end of the day, when I devote another twenty minutes to doing my best to recognize that all my experiences were positive lessons that God would have me learn, even though they may not have seemed so.

Next, I make a prayer of thanking God for my blessings, for all the blessings that were bestowed on me. I then express my willingness to have a peaceful night and to walk along with God in my sleep.

Patricia Norris

HEALING: WHAT WE CAN LEARN FROM CHILDREN

Patricia Norris, Ph.D., is clinical director of the Biofeedback and Psycho-physiology Center at the Menninger Clinic in Topeka, Kansas. She is a therapist, researcher, and teacher of self-regulation of mind/body processes. She is coauthor (with Garrett Porter) of I Choose Life: The Dynamics of Visualization and Biofeedback.

I n addition to the underlying commonalities shared by all therapies and therapists, there is another golden thread that represents the other half of the equation in a healing process: the self-healing abilities of the client.

In my work with psychophysiologic therapy, the goal is self-regulation, self-healing, by the client. The therapist's role is to teach the patient to heal, to be both coach and cheerleader in this process. So the qualities the client brings to the treatment process, or acquires during therapy, are of central importance to the ongoing process and the outcome.

What are the qualities and conditions of mind that promote positive outcomes, a healing relationship between the mind and the body's healing resources? Recently interest has grown in exploring qualities that promote wellness, that keep us healthy or contribute to healing or to survival of catastrophic disease.

In my own work, while observing child clients, I became interested in significant personal factors in healing and how to evoke them. Children show great ability to enter the healing process and to learn self-regulation. Almost invariably, as every therapist who uses biofeedback-assisted self-regulation with children knows, they are able to warm their hands (increase blood flow to their hands) readily, just by thinking about it.

Children, who are naturally open, accepting, trusting, enthusiastic, nonjudgmental, and ready to learn, can be an example for us of how to approach healing. We can look to their strengths to find evidence of a golden thread of healing, a readiness for transformation. Children are in the process of learning everything: to walk, run, speak, ride a bike, read, write; in other words, how to handle their bodies, their language, and culture. They are open to learning and expect to be able to accomplish what they set out to do. If you tell them they can do something, they don't question it. If you say, "When you turn this knob, the TV will come on," they say, "Okay," and they turn the knob. Tell them that they can make their hands warm, that they can send more blood to their toes, or that they can send white blood cells to fight their tumors, and they say, "Okay," and do it. One task is the same as another.

This was my strategy with Garrett, my first cancer client, a child with a brain tumor. I learned so much from him about the healing process; indeed, all my clients have been my teachers. Garrett learned to warm his hands, then his feet, then any part of his body to which he turned his attention. He learned some heart-rate control and excellent control of his electrodermal response. Biofeedback provided convincing proof that control was indeed within his power. Because he had seen that he could send blood wherever he wanted in his body, it was not hard for him to believe that he could also send white cells to affect immune-system action.

"Let me do it myself" is a familiar refrain to anyone who knows children. As soon as they are able, and even before, they are eager to do things on their own. This eagerness can be especially important for children with catastrophic illness such as severe burns or cancer. The treatments they must have are often traumatic, and despite the best efforts of all concerned, children are sometimes deeply scarred emotionally by their experiences. They have a harder time than adults in understanding how something painful and scary can help them or ultimately make them feel better, when the more immediate effects are so unpleasant. Their capacity for self-regulation can stand them in

good stead in facing difficult treatments. If they can feel like participants in their own healing, finding a way to ameliorate some of their
discomfort and anxiety, the results can be profoundly positive.

As Tommy, who had undergone a series of harsh treatments for
Hodgkin's disease, told me: "One thing I don't think they put enough
emphasis on is the need for understanding and the importance of
helping a patient release anger. I believe the mind is what cured me,
but anger swelled up in me from my cancer, and all the effort was on
making me physically better. There was no relief from the anger. It
was, 'Well, we have to help you live!'

"It's harder for a young kid to have a clear concept of what
you're doing with the chemotherapy. In biofeedback I *knew* what we
were doing to get the mind over the cancer. It was a painful but
growing experience. Now I think in terms of living a lifetime."

Tommy did withstand his painful treatments more easily and
more positively with the self-regulation he was learning from biofeedback and visualization.

Children have the ability to accept their own power and responsibility without blame or guilt. To adults, the idea that we can assume
responsibility for our wellness often suggests that we must be causing
our own illness. Our self-doubt says, "If I am responsible, then I am
to blame." Of course, no one chooses to be ill on purpose or in any
conscious way. Children accept learning to make themselves well with
no more guilt than if they were learning to write or talk.

There is a world of difference between the fixing of blame and
the accepting of responsibility. The fact that we can assume responsibility and begin to take charge of our health and our lives is good
news. As Elmer Green has pointed out, if there is such a thing as
psychosomatic illness (and no one doubts it), there must also be such
a thing as psychosomatic health. If we can make ourselves sick (unin-
tentionally), then we can—with intentionality—make ourselves well.
It is precisely this acceptance of responsibility that starts the real
transformative process of healing. It represents change from a "victim
consciousness" to a sense of empowerment.

We often think of people who are ill as "victims" of disease, and
this reinforces their sense of helplessness. An important part of our
work is to give adults who need healing the sense of empowerment
that children naturally have. It is the opposite of helplessness: it is a
sense of one's own potential to be, to do, and to feel. One young girl
who had Hodgkin's disease told me, "The way I changed, even more
than getting over the cancer, is that I like myself better now."

Developmentally, children are in a state of close integration of conscious and unconscious processes. This is one of the things that make them such good learners. If you go to a foreign country with children four or five years old, you will notice them soon speaking the new language like natives. Learning takes place on several levels of consciousness at once.

Now we are discovering that adults also can learn things like language rapidly, by deliberately emulating the state of consciousness children are in most of the time, with techniques such as those employed by superlearning and twilight learning. One aim of therapy is to access the unconscious in order to increase conscious control of it. This is what self-regulation and voluntary control of internal states accomplish physiologically, with profound psychological effects as well.

Clients often come to a healing situation with diminished self-esteem and a diminished sense of self-mastery. To the extent that they are diminished, learning cannot take place. Children, if they receive normal and loving care, naturally have good self-esteem and little experience with failure. Self-discovery is exciting for them. Children are able to confront problems that often astound an adult.

Several children with whom I've worked have had out-of-body experiences that they simply took at face value. They do not worry about whether an experience conflicts with some belief system. Garrett told me, "My inner body comes out at night and floats around in the living room." Later, when Garrett and I were talking and I wanted to refer to his more permanent self, I said, "You know, Garrett, it's like your inner body . . ." He looked at me seriously and said, "That's my true self, you know." I was quite surprised; he must have been speaking from some deep place of wisdom.

Children also confront death more easily and naturally than adults. I find that this ability is important to the healing process. Everyone can benefit from coming to terms with death. An openness to the possibility of death helps children enter the healing process as an adventure and see getting well as a possibility but not the only outcome necessary for healing to take place. There can be a healing death as well. Fear of death can create a self-fulfilling prophecy. It is important for patients to feel that death is not an enemy. Children move closer or further away from death in an easy flow. Children are naturally able to live in the present, to "be here now," to exist easily in a state of being that adults often have to work hard to relearn through meditation, therapy, or some other conscious effort.

Another factor that helps people to heal is being of service. I see in children a natural empathy; they want to help each other. They have an ability to be even-handed toward themselves and others, like living on both sides of the golden rule—to love others as oneself and to love oneself as others.

Of course, the therapist needs to believe in the client's potential to heal himself. A belief that what one is attempting is possible, even though not guaranteed, is essential. Negative beliefs and self-doubts impose unnecessary limitations. Positive expectation, together with positive experience of control, eliminates doubts. These hopes come easily for children.

Fortunately, we can change how we perceive ourselves and how we relate to the stressors in our lives. We can acquire the skills and the resources to deal with stress as a challenge and as a learning opportunity. Learning to self-regulate our responses to stress gradually leads us to meet challenge with a sense of energy and exhilaration rather than worry and despair. This change of attitude can have a powerful healing effect.

It is natural for our bodies to heal. The aspiration to improve ourselves, to reach out constantly toward a greater goal, is exemplified by children. It is available to all of us if we are willing to recapture those strengths that are part of our natural heritage—our potential to be well, our potential for choice, self-healing, self-direction, and self-mastery.

Part Seven

CONSCIOUSNESS AND THE HEALING RESPONSE

Complete health and awakening are really the same.
Tarthang Tulku

Healing goes far beyond the confines of the physical body. It occurs when we tap into our own inner resources rather than look for external intervention. It is the inner connection with that part of ourselves that is already healed; a retraining of our minds to accept the flow and ever-changing conditions of life. With intention and practice we can learn to control our minds. With this control comes the deepest kind of healing, which is victory over suffering.

The contributors here explain how a "quiet mind" shows us the nature of change and impermanence. Through our quietness, we begin to accept our own suffering and pain. We discover that surrender to our sickness is often our only route through it.

As we quietly learn to accept all aspects of life, we awaken to the totality of ourselves. Disease and suffering arise from a mind that is unwhole, that is filled with confusion and despair. To be "healed" means to restore oneself to a place in which the mind is at peace.

Joan Halifax

THE MIND
OF HEALING

*Joan Halifax, Ph.D., is an anthropologist who has worked with shamans
and healers the world over. She is president of the Ojai Foundation in
Ojai, California, and a founder of The Foundation School. She has
authored* Shamanic Voices *and* Shaman, The Wounded Healer.
*She is a practicing Buddhist. Her essay was inspired by Richard Baker-
roshi's teachings on the five levels of practice.*

There is a Zen story that opens an avenue of inquiry into the
location of the source of suffering and sanity. Many years ago, a
monk in a Zen monastery in Japan was struggling with his meditation
practice. Each time he sat to meditate, he saw a giant spider threaten-
ing him. After experiencing much anxiety and losing much sleep, he
finally decided to kill the creature.

As he was walking toward the meditation hall with a big knife
in his hand, his teacher saw him and asked what he intended to do.
The young man explained his plight. The master listened attentively
and recommended a strategy to the young monk. He told him first to
get his calligraphy brush and carefully paint a cross on the spider's
belly, then to put the knife into the intersection of the cross on the
following day.

The monk entered the meditation hall with his brush and ink.
When the spider appeared, he carefully painted its belly. Feeling quite
satisfied, he bowed and left the meditation hall—and discovered on
the front of his robes a huge painted X. His laughter was heard
everywhere.

This monk had placed the monster somewhere outside of himself. To another, the monster could well appear within. In the practice of mindfulness, we are encouraged to notice that the mind has a strong tendency to create love and hate, birth and death, sickness and sanity, even monsters and magic. It is taught by culture and society to play hide-and-seek with itself, a game of forgetfulness in the constant flow of the diversionary activity of mind, feelings, and physical sensations, whether pleasant, unpleasant, or neutral. These obsessions drive us into patterns of greater or lesser suffering and illness that are difficult to escape.

Buddhism and shamanism offer training in the art of lucidity, awareness, or mindfulness. This cultivation of awareness is rooted in the ground of motivation or intent. This is where healing begins and where suffering begins to cease. Ultimately, the experience of intent needs to be completely penetrating for the body/mind to reorganize itself out of its pattern of suffering. The unfolding of intent occurs within the experience of the individual becoming genuinely familiar with the content and movement of the mind. In Buddhism, this can arise through the practice of meditation or mindfulness.

In meditation practice, we discover that new realms open for us. In entering the Zendo, or meditation room, we have chosen to be physically still and silent. We have left the activity of our ordinary lives and are in voluntary seclusion. From one point of view, entering the Zendo and entering the hospital are not so different. In both cases, a cure for suffering is sought. Like the Native American apprentice who prays for vision on the mountaintop, the meditator chooses sacred seclusion. The hospital patient, however, usually has not made that choice consciously. Rather, illness has made it necessary to withdraw from ordinary life. Yet in each case there is withdrawal from the activities and social domain of daily life and a retreat into solitude.

In meditation practice, we begin to quiet ourselves, to calm ourselves. In stopping our usual activity, we notice how the relentless flow of the mind drives us. Through the experience of stilling and calming, we begin to get a glimmer of the nature of change, of impermanence. Later, through physically stilling ourselves, we become internally quieter as our capacity for self-observation deepens.

The next realm of practice begins to open as we continue to sit through the question of intent. When we have ceased to wrestle with time and have approached the border of accepting the usefulness of "non-doing," the spaciousness of patience begins to open before us. As we accept and surrender to practice, we also begin to accept our own suffering and, in deeper states of absorption, our death. In the experience of healing, the surrender to pain and suffering is often the route through it. Here also we can experience the surrender to healer and teacher. Through the experience of surrender, we begin to work more concretely with impermanence. We accept practice as a way to approach positively the experience of change. One student noted, "Change is inevitable; growth is optional." Accepting practice as medicine to cure suffering, and intending practice to foster pure understanding, we find that pure awareness opens the way for these conditions to actually happen.

One of the most important effects of mindfulness practice is that it can produce a synchronization of mind and body through the union of breath and awareness, and then of mind and body with reality. Here we find strong evidence of the golden thread that unites healing methods of all types. It has been repeatedly observed that illness and suffering flow through the gap in the mind/body relationship. When there is no synchronization of mind, body, and the outside world, when there is an absence of awareness of the interconnectedness of inside with outside, the experience of alienation pervades the mind.

The meditator deepens concentration through a more vivid connection with practice. The observer becomes one with breath, with fewer mental diversions arising. The body and mind ride the ebb and flow of breath. The mind and body begin to recognize each other; they have long been partners but turned their backs on each other long ago. The mind began to push the body about like an animal trainer who does not consider the well-being of his charge. The body's desire or aversion began to create patterns of craving or dislike in the mind. The reunion between body and mind is sewn with the thread of breath in the light of concentration.

The next realm of practice relates to the experience of insight, realization, or understanding. Until now, the mind has been ruled by conditions. When the mind's capacity for discernment awakens, it is possible to perceive, realize, or understand directly. In the case of healing, realization of the source, purpose, and cure of illness arises when the culturally conditioned mind has lost its grip on the deeper mindfield. Understanding and reorganizing entrenched patterns can occur through conditionless cognition or direct perception. This is the experience of "stopping the world" or stopping the mind. The mind is still for change. In shamanism, this is called seeing; in Buddhism, mindfulness.

Mindfulness practice takes on a social dimension when the meditator sees clearly the suffering of the world. In Mahayana Buddhism, there is a great emphasis on doing what is correct not only for oneself but also for others. The well-known promise, "I vow to attain enlightenment in order to save all sentient beings from suffering," becomes a reference point in the direction of sanity for the Buddhist. This aspect of practice takes us into the marketplace. The emphasis is on the experience of engagement. Here we find healers, shamans, teachers, and peacemakers, those who have made a commitment to transforming social institutions that are fostering disease, and to helping individuals, cultures, and environments that are suffering.

Engagement practice indicates that we have developed the capacity to act with complete appropriateness in the face of all eventualities and to work with each moment in an enlightened way. In Zen, we often hear, "When you are hungry, eat; when you are tired, sleep." Do only what is correct and necessary. This is being in harmony with the world. When we have wrestled with the enemies of our own lives and minds, making them allies, we then have the potential to befriend the enemies of the world. This is called reconciliation, or peace.

Mindfulness, then, belongs in the field of social as well as personal action. It is the ground on which compassion is born. This compassion is not the self-aggrandizing messianic form of saviorism. It is sober and even ruthless, precise and economical. It is context-sensitive and aware of consequences. Often it is invisible.

And this leads us to the ultimate realm to be realized in practice —that of secret practice. Here we have fully realized ordinary mind, ordinary life. Mind, body, and reality have become one. Big Mind penetrates each moment, each thing. No obstacle, no enlightenment, no death, no big deal.

In conclusion, mindfulness can be seen as the golden thread or substrate of healing. It can be viewed, in fact, as synonymous with healing. Disease and suffering arise from a mind that is divided by passion, hatred, and confusion. To be healed means to have been restored to one's original nature, when mind, body, and the world are one.

Ram Dass

THE INTUITIVE HEART

Ram Dass (Richard Alpert, Ph.D.) has been one of the most influential leaders of the consciousness movement since the early 1960s. He is the author of several popular books, including Be Here Now *and* Grist for the Mill *(with Stephen Levine). He is chairman of the Seva Foundation, a nonprofit organization dedicated to the relief of suffering throughout the world.*

Whether our methods involve words or touch, meditations or medicines, our techniques and interventions are vehicles of transmission. What they transmit is an environment in which healing can occur. Just as in a garden, we do not "grow" flowers; rather, we create the conditions in which flowers can grow.

The conditions for healing involve faith in the possibility that healing can occur, and resonance with the deeper and wiser parts of the self where healing *is.* In this realm of deeper truth, we can find access to the laws and harmonies that underlie form (the Way of things as described in the Tao Te Ching). Here we comprehend the perfection in which the experience of the need and desire to be healed is itself part of that perfection. Resting in that deeper truth, we are at once healed. The symptom or negative state may or may not disappear, but in the deeper context and faith, suffering is no more. Suffering cannot be taken away, it can only be relinquished.

When asked his message, Mahatma Gandhi replied, "My life is my message." So, too, for us; what we do conveys what we are. If we are to be an environment for healing, a provider of heart-to-heart resuscitation, we must examine the extent of our own faith and resonance. And where it is as yet undeveloped, we must cultivate it. This is the work on ourselves that simultaneously frees us from suffering and allows us to be present where healing in others occurs.

Learning to hear, really hear, is a root component of this work. We hear what is, both in the depths of our own being and in the nature of the suffering of another. Because "the truth waits for eyes unclouded by longing," we cultivate equanimity in order to hear. The knowledge required for our specific techniques or methods must have been absorbed so thoroughly that we can transcend what we know in order to listen quietly and freshly, trusting our own wisdom.

Hearing ourselves allows us to witness the way in which we become entrapped in our ego's conviction that it does the healing. As we relinquish this attachment of mind, the way in which the universe works through us becomes clearer. Similarly, we witness how attached our minds are to the fruits of our actions. A wise practitioner lets go of this attachment as well. He or she acts impeccably, and then trusts in the wisdom inherent in the universe to determine the outcome.

We are healed into truth, so truth is a cornerstone we must tend to scrupulously. A healer must be ready, willing, and able to share his or her own truth. Which of the many truths available to us that we share from moment to moment is a function of what we hear when we have learned to listen?

In the ultimate depth of being, we find ourselves no longer separate but, rather, part of the unity of the universe. That unity includes the sufferer and the suffering, and the healer and that which heals. Therefore, all acts of healing are ultimately our selves healing our Self.

Larry Dossey

MIND BEYOND BODY

Larry Dossey, M.D., is former chief of staff at Medical City Dallas Hospital and a well-known authority in alternative approaches to healing. He is the author of Space, Time, and Medicine; Beyond Illness; *and* Mind Beyond Body *(in press).*

I t is possible to focus on the differences separating the myriad approaches to healing that have surfaced throughout human history, and there is much to be gained by this approach. But the differences seem to speak for themselves, for many of them are obvious: We can see the gigantic distinctions in techniques employed by an aboriginal shaman and a modern internist. What is not obvious is the invisible unifying factor that pervades healing from antiquity to the present day, overriding the obvious differences. This unifying factor can be singled out as mind or consciousness.

How does mind enter into healing, and how does it unify what healers have done since time immemorial?

To get an answer we have to go beyond the common-sense view of reality that dominates our Western way of defining the world, and be willing to entertain the possibility that things may not be the way they seem. When certain cultures have allowed themselves to believe that the senses may not tell all, new visions of the world have opened up. The resulting world view can be described as "layered," or ordered according to some kind of hierarchy. In this arrangement, some layers of reality are usually perceived to be more real or more significant than others.

When human beings have taken such a hierarchical view of the way the world works, mind and consciousness are invariably placed near the top. As one descends in the scale of order to the "lower" levels—down past human beings, animals, and plants, to rocks, molecules, and atoms—the degree of consciousness diminishes. So in the hierarchical view the entire world may be alive with mind, although of different degrees. Mind is spread throughout the world from this perspective, which is to say that it is nonlocal, not confined to certain points.

In our own culture, however, we have said exactly the opposite: Mind is local. It is confined to the brain and is merely a product of the brain's anatomy, physiology, and chemistry. Destruction of the brain, therefore, means destruction of the mind. Furthermore, the local approach to the mind means that minds are multiple—one mind per each of the four and a half billion human brains on our planet.

This local approach has had great appeal in our culture and, of course, much evidence favors it. But this way of looking at the mind breaks down when we examine the way minds actually behave.

In fact, the mind steadfastly refuses to behave locally, as contemporary scientific evidence is beginning to show. We now know, for instance, that brainlike tissue is found throughout the body. Receptor sites for chemical endorphins have been discovered in many places outside the brain, in the gastrointestinal tract and in certain types of white blood cells. And endorphins are actually made at sites distant from the brain. So, even from the conservative perspective of modern neurochemistry, it is difficult if not impossible to follow a strictly local view of the brain.

Furthermore, today the mind seems even more nonlocal. Not only does it appear to have burst the bounds of the brain to invade the entire body, but it seems to have escaped the body altogether. There is much data suggesting that the mind is at large in the world, that it is not *in a place* at all. Among the strongest evidence for this is a series of experiments done in the past few years at Princeton University's Engineering Anomalies Research Laboratory by Professor Robert G. Jahn and Brenda Dunne (see *Margins of Reality,* New York: Harcourt Brace Jovanovich, 1987).

In a computer-controlled experiment, Jahn and Dunne have shown that minds can communicate complex messages in detail across enormous distances. It seems to make no difference if the individuals are separated by one block or if they are on opposite sides of the earth. The messages get through, sometimes in astonishing detail. Moreover, neither does *temporal* separation seem to be a factor. The information sometimes gets through to the receiver up to three days before it is sent! And this talent is not just possessed by a few skilled subjects; ordinary people can do it as well.

These findings are reinforced by the careful studies of cardiologist Randy Byrd of San Francisco General Hospital showing the distant effects of prayer on critically ill patients. His research showed that it seemed to make no difference whether the person praying was next door to the patient or thousands of miles away.

Local views of the mind cannot explain these findings. We are free, of course, to discard this information and say that it is wrong or fraudulent (as critics frequently maintain). But if we try to explain them, these data lead to a different picture of consciousness than our local, physically based, here-and-now view. In the alternate view the mind is nonlocal, unconfined to points in space or time, and immaterial.

The picture does not stop here. If minds are not in a place in space or time, then they are unbounded; if unbounded, then they are not separate. This means they cannot be individual, as we have always thought. True, mind may act through individual brains, just as a radio signal can act through a receiver. But that isn't the complete story. Fundamentally, mind must be one, not many.

This view of the unitary nature of the mind, which has much modern evidence to support it, leads to a new view of healing. It suggests that there is only one nonlocal mind at work in the healing process. The minds of all healers are one, united nonlocally beyond space and time. This one mind envelops the patient as well. In this view, all therapy is self-directed, for there really is no "other" who exists outside the therapist. Accordingly, healers never act alone. They act in concert as a consequence of the nonlocal nature of the mind.

As we think about new models of human consciousness and apply them to our daily experiences, we must continually try to avoid oversimplification. There has been a regrettable tendency to say that, if all minds are one, then all illness is one. But this is patently not so. It is your leg that is broken, not mine; it is my cancer that is being treated, not yours. We should not forget, as we observed above, that there is a hierarchy that is part of the world, and that distinctions are created in this manifest world through this ordering principle. So some processes seem more or less mental, while others seem more or less physical. If we forget these distinctions we will wind up in greater confusion than before.

True, the body is related to mind, but this does not mean they are the same, blurred together in some indistinguishable goo. Bodies incontrovertibly have a way of manifesting *as if* they are separate; they break down *as if* they are machines; and they can sometimes be repaired *as if* they are machines. If we fail to recognize this fact, we run the risk of neglecting many valuable therapies and of reinventing "medical" approaches such as sympathetic magic, in which I treat your broken arm by putting the cast on my arm. These therapies have a fatal flaw: they don't work.

So, in our enthusiasm for the role of the mind in healing, we must take care not to abandon the physically based therapies that are right and humane, always recalling that the world, including the body, does have a way of manifesting in the most obdurate physical ways, and that when it does so, physically based therapies may be appropriate.

As our models of health and illness change toward a recognition of the role of consciousness, we need to remember the nonlocal nature of mind. Unfortunately this caution is frequently thrown to the winds. Even among the growing number of those who recognize the role of the mind in healing, the emphasis is usually on teaching a patient to use the *individual* mind to overcome an *individual* health problem. The unitary nature of the mind is almost always forgotten. But we cannot have it both ways. We cannot remain ego-centered individuals and know the full healing power of the one mind at the same time.

The contemporary Sufi master Pir Vilayat Khan has said, "The assumption of being an individual is our greatest limitation" (Gary Doore, "The Dynamics of Transformation," in *The American Theosophist,* Spring 1986). It is a distortion of our nonlocal Self—who we really are. With the cult of the individual comes the intensification of illness, suffering, and death. We may search for cures that focus solely on the individual person ad infinitum, even "mind cures." But no matter how sophisticated they may be, they will always prove insufficient, because the central problem—our belief that we are local, limited, individual creatures—will remain untouched. For this disease there is only one cure—the Great Cure, which comes about when we wake up to the nonlocal, unbounded nature of the Self.

Harold Bloomfield

THE HEALING SILENCE

Harold Bloomfield, M.D., is a practicing psychiatrist and director of psychiatry, psychotherapy, and health training at the North County Holistic Health Center in Del Mar, California. His best-selling books include How to Survive the Loss of a Love, TM: Discovering Inner Energy and Overcoming Stress, *and* How to Enjoy the Love of Your Life.

M edical professionals have long recognized that silence plays an important role in healing. Bed rest, for example, is the usual prescription for many illnesses, from the common cold to myocardial infarction. The more ill you are, the more your doctor will insist that you be quiet and rest.

But despite this age-old appreciation of the value of silence, medical and psychological researchers and practitioners until recently paid scant attention to states of *internal silence.* It is my belief that the timeless quality of silence is so important that we can call it one of the common denominators of successful healing.

There are many reasons for the neglect of silence in our Western culture. Perhaps the greatest is our belief that a successful person is a dynamic individual who works hard, enjoys life fully, and can withstand the pressure and tension of a fast-paced life. To many people, inner tranquility suggests a lack of drive, a dull personality, and an inability to compete. Passion, joy, and all the other emotions that make living vibrant are thought to be antithetical to inner silence.

This bias against inner silence is a serious mistake. To appreciate how inner silence can strengthen total healing and well-being, we must look at the concept of stress. Though the term is often used loosely, it has a specific scientific meaning. Dr. Hans Selye, a pioneer on the subject, defined it as "the body's nonspecific response to any demand made on it." Bodily changes accompanying stress may include muscular tension, increased heart rate, accelerated breathing, sweating, and anxiety.

Inner silence has profound effects on both the body and mind. One experiences a state of deep rest, marked by decreases in heartbeat rate, oxygen consumption, perspiration, muscle tension, blood pressure, and levels of stress hormones. One also achieves a state of heightened mental clarity and emotional ease. Whereas stress saps vitality, silence restores it. Whereas stress lowers resistance to disease, silence raises it.

The physiological changes that neutralize the effects of stress also affect emotional health. Inner silence reduces anxiety, tension, irritability, chronic fatigue, and depression. The positive feelings that accompany such reductions add noticeably to personality development. Self-esteem grows, sociability develops, and doubts and insecurities fade.

Inner silence is crucial to health. Periods of solitude are essential to the continued vitality of the highly creative and self-actualizing person. Studies show that such people almost invariably make time in their busy schedules for some quiet solitude. At the level of deep inner silence, the psyche can heal itself quietly and naturally without having to verbalize or examine long-buried emotional traumas.

Cultivation of inner silence has long been recognized in many cultures as a cornerstone of spiritual growth. Meditation, after all, has been passed down for thousands of years, not primarily as a means to better health, but rather as an instrument to achieve the heights of spiritual development and awareness. Deep in meditation, the inner silence can be so profound that one gains a state of expanded awareness, recognizing one's innermost self as distinct from one's body, mind, and feelings. This experience is deeply satisfying and produces lasting positive effects.

There are many important factors in the process of healing. However, I can think of no more important aspect than the quality of inner silence. As therapists of all types become more aware of this powerful state, great strides will be made in the science of healing.

Deepak Chopra

THE SPELL
OF MORTALITY

*Deepak Chopra, M.D., is president of the American Association of
Ayurvedic Medicine, former assistant clinical professor of sociomedical
sciences at Boston University School of Medicine, and former chief of staff
at New England Memorial Hospital. He is the author of* Creating
Health: Beyond Prevention, Toward Perfection *and* Return of
the Rishi: A Doctor's Search for the Ultimate Healer.

Several patients have taught me that the healing process is still not
fully appreciated. The most memorable of these was a middle-aged
woman who came to me about ten years ago complaining of severe
abdominal pains and jaundice. Believing that she was suffering from
gallstones, I had her admitted for surgery. When she was opened up,
it was found that she had no gallstones but a large malignant tumor
that had spread to her liver, with scattered pockets of cancer throughout the abdominal cavity.

Judging the case inoperable, her surgeons closed the incision
without taking any further action. Because the woman's daughter
pleaded with me not to tell her mother the truth, I informed my
patient that the gallstones had been removed successfully. I rational-
ized that her family would break the news to her in time, and that at
best she had only a few months to live—at least she could spend them
with peace of mind.

Eight months later I was astonished to see the woman in my
office. She had returned for a routine physical exam, which revealed
no jaundice, pain, or detectable signs of cancer. Only a year later did

she confess anything unusual to me. She said, "Doctor, I was so sure I had cancer then that when it turned out to be just gallstones, I told myself I would never be sick another day in my life." Her cancer never recurred.

This case has led me to consider that modern medicine has restricted itself to an extremely narrow view of healing. The question we should ask is not "What is healing?" It has always been known that healing is a process controlled by nature. The crucial question is, rather, "Does healing have any natural limit?" So far as I know, the answer is no.

Because we limit ourselves to a set scheme of medicine, with its "normal" diagnoses, treatments, and expectations, we suppose that nature accepts our boundaries as normal. Nature obviously does not agree.

When we say that no one knows the cure for cancer, we are telling a half-truth. The way that this woman was cured, from within herself, is *the* cure for cancer. It came about when a radical shift took place somewhere inside her physiology, yet the exact location of this shift opens up profound mysteries. It defies current medical wisdom to answer even the most basic question: Was the shift in her mind, in her body, or both?

To find out, Western medicine has begun to gradually move away from drugs and surgery, the mainstays of every physician's practice. An amorphous, often perplexing field loosely known as "mind-body medicine" is arising. The move away from the old, mechanistic system of medicine was almost a forced one, because our old reliance on the stability of the physical body had begun to crumble.

Mind-body medicine makes many doctors extremely uneasy because it is more a concept than a field. Given a choice between a concept and a chemical, a doctor will trust the chemical. Penicillin, digitalis, aspirin, and Valium do not need any new ideas on the patient's part (or the doctor's) to be effective. The problem comes in when the chemical is not effective.

Up-to-date surveys taken in England and America have shown that as many as 80 percent of patients feel that their underlying complaint, their reason for going to the doctor, was not satisfactorily resolved when they left the doctor's office. Classic studies going back to the end of World War II showed that patients left the Yale Medical School hospital feeling sicker than the day they arrived. These are paralleled by similar studies showing that patients with psychiatric complaints improved more while they were on the waiting list to see a psychiatrist than after they actually saw one. So the situation isn't simply one of exchanging a body doctor for a head doctor.

A miracle cure throws into high relief the need to reexamine medicine's basic concepts. Our current logic of healing can lead to impressive, or at least adequate, results, as when we use penicillin to wipe out a broad range of infectious diseases. But nature's logic of healing can be awe-inspiring. Many physicians have stood in wonder witnessing such cures without having a clue as to how to explain them; the standard term for them is "spontaneous remission," a convenient tag that says little more than that the patient recovered by himself.

Medicine has been blind in thinking that matter is more powerful than mind. Now, in an attempt to overcome this blindness, curious and adventurous doctors have flocked to experiment with mind-body innovations over the last decade, from biofeedback and hypnotism to visualization and behavior modification. The results across the board have been amorphous and hard to interpret. In 1985, an in-depth study of 300 alternative approaches to cancer discovered that they gave a measure of comfort and relief to patients, but the remission rates were not radically different from those in standard therapy.

There are other problems that run deeper than inconsistent results: The mind-body field continues to be plagued by an inability to rigorously prove its basic tenet, that the mind influences the body toward either health or disease. It seems utterly self-evident that sick people and healthy people do not share the same state of mind, but the causal connection is elusive.

The intricacies of the mind-body relation are not easily solved. If we ask why a positive mind cannot be easily correlated with good health—it appears to be one of the most obvious facts of life—the answer has to do with what we mean by mind in the first place. This is not a philosophical question but a practical one. If a patient comes in with cancer, is his mental state judged by how he feels on the day of the diagnosis, or long before, or long afterward? Do we accept his conscious thoughts, emotions, beliefs, desires, wishes, and fantasies as his mind, or are we to look into the dark unconscious?

We will not answer these questions, I believe, until we rejoin the perennial traditions of mankind. Because Western medicine assumes that a person is a physical machine who happens to think, we find ourselves out on a limb, a naked spur of history. The great traditions of wisdom, embracing medicine, philosophy, psychology, and religion, have all believed exactly the opposite: We are thoughts that have learned to create a physical machine. As a basis for healing, we must deal with the body if a patient is in dire need. But over the course of a lifetime, what shapes every human being, for good or ill, is his overall, or holistic, status, and that is rooted in consciousness.

My particular interest has turned to Ayurveda, India's ancient "science of life." (My understanding and practice of Ayurveda owes everything to Maharishi Mahesh Yogi, who is responsible for the modern revival of Ayurveda and for restoring its most effective techniques.)

Ayurveda survives today as basically an extensive system of natural medicine. However, when it originated more than 5000 years ago, Ayurveda was cognized in the minds of the ancient Vedic seers, or rishis, as a completely fixed, stable body of knowledge dealing with human life on the basis of cosmic life. A famous verse from Ayurveda says:

> As is the human body, so is the cosmic body.
> As is the human mind, so is the cosmic mind.
> As is the microcosm, so is the macrocosm.
> As is the atom, so is the universe.

Whatever we may think from our local perspective, this is the classic statement, the mainstream of human understanding. Quantum physics would have to agree that the human body, like all complex physical structures, is created from invisible fluctuations in nature's fundamental energy fields. This body that seems so solid is really made of energy waves, or vibrations, and even if we could get close enough to inspect the spots and dots of matter that whirl at lightning speed around the atomic nucleus, the void between them is as empty as intergalactic space.

What keeps this void together? Without calling it a mind, physics has come to admit that an infinitely powerful, orderly, all-embracing eternal principle has operated since the first billionth of a second after the Big Bang, shaping this immense void into stars, planets, life forms, and mankind. Ayurveda holds that this principle is nothing other than consciousness and is perfectly reflected in our own consciousness. In one mode, consciousness expresses itself as matter, in another as mind, with infinite gradations in between.

Consciousness can move or be still, but it always remains in control. Think of our own DNA, which is just as much an expression of knowledge as of matter. DNA controls life from the wings without ever stepping center-stage. In one mode it sits fixed in its place within the cell's nucleus. In another mode, it creates RNA to produce proteins. Eventually, as the proteins give rise to enzymes, we are dealing with an enormously complex living structure, but all its parts are still connected to the basic nature of DNA—not to its atoms or molecules, which sit at a distance, but to the pure knowledge DNA exhibits.

When a messenger molecule, like the hormone thyroxin, floats down the bloodstream and attaches itself to a receptor on the cell wall, we are witnessing one aspect of DNA interacting with another. The receptor is like an ear awaiting a message, and the hormone is the answer. But taken all in all, the whole process is intelligence talking to itself. This simple idea is enough to depose many outworn assumptions in medicine—the assumption that only the brain thinks, that mind is not part of matter, that activity in physiology can sometimes be random.

Once we see ourselves as creations of intelligence, then we must admit that we are self-created. Actually, we are in the process of self-creating, because intelligence never ceases to communicate with itself. The blood is not a chemical soup; it is a multilane freeway in which thousands of messages, conveyed by hormones, neuropeptides, immune cells, and enzymes, are forever traveling, each intent on some mission, each capable of maintaining its own integrity as an impulse of intelligence.

Medicine is desperately in search of new metaphors to get us beyond the huge obstacles that still face us, such as cancer and AIDS. Ayurveda suggests a metaphor that is simple but at the same time incredibly powerful: Life is like a tree, and its root is consciousness. Therefore, once we tend the root, the tree as a whole will be healthy. Nature controls healing from this deeper level already, for every cell participates in the body's inner intelligence, responding to the patient's thoughts, emotions, desires, beliefs, and self-image.

Mind always has some physical correlate. Every physician in practice has seen people who died, apparently not from a disease but from a diagnosis. I once treated a man in his fifties who had lived comfortably for five years with a coin-sized lesion in his lung that was growing very slowly. After reexamining his old chest X rays, I told him that the lesion was consistent with a diagnosis of lung cancer. He was distraught to hear this. Despite having had no overt symptoms in the past, he began to cough up blood within a month, and within three months he was dead.

Nature did not put up a wall between mind and body. Our own boundaries are real only because we have conditioned ourselves to believe in them. We are prisoners of our own conditioning, who need healing in order to be released from the spells we have cast, spells of disease and illness, ignorance and suffering. The chief aim of Ayurveda is to break the spell of ignorance and then allow nature itself to do the healing. Breaking centuries of conditioning is at once very easy and very difficult. It is difficult in the ordinary waking state, which creates one boundary after another, but easy in the state of pure consciousness, or unbounded awareness.

The ancient Ayurvedic rishis assumed that human beings would always cherish their birthright of unbounded consciousness. A famous Vedic verse says, "Of bliss these creatures are born, in bliss they are sustained, and to bliss they merge again." The ground of a healthy, whole life is this pure form of consciousness, called bliss or *Ananda*. Bliss is the closest thing to a life force that nature has provided. Insofar as a patient can be put back into contact with it, he will experience the rise of healing within himself. Inasmuch as he is a prisoner of fragmented values, he will be a prey to disease, infirmity, and all the other ills cast by the spell of mortality.

I cannot envision a healthy future until the spell is broken and we understand once again what the mainstream of human wisdom has always taught: The field of human life is immortal. It is the field of the universe localized within ourselves.

Part Eight

HEALING AS OUR BIRTHRIGHT

We attend in silence and in joy.
This is the day when healing comes to us.
This is the day when separation ends,
and we remember Who we really are.

A Course in Miracles

Healing is more than a reversal of disease or injury. In fact, many healings are superficial because their focus is limited to the physical body. The reason we take birth is to rediscover the deeper, wiser parts of ourselves. By becoming aware that our lives are a continual process of healing, we can learn to come to peace with any illness or injury that may manifest.

Each contributor in this section believes that healing is a process of reconnecting with that part of us that always was, always is, and always will be. We take birth as an opportunity to work through the issues that develop in our lives; to make peace with and come to terms with who we are. The golden thread of healing, in this sense, is seen as a process of personal transformation, a process of becoming one with ourselves. Our lives are vehicles to connect with the childlike qualities we are born with, which are uninjured, innocent, and whole.

Joan Borysenko

REMOVING BARRIERS TO THE PEACEFUL CORE

Joan Borysenko, Ph.D., is former director of the Mind/Body Clinic at New England Deaconess Hospital, Harvard Medical School. Trained as both a cell biologist and as a psychologist, she is also a teacher of yoga and meditation. Author of Minding the Body, Mending the Mind, *she is now president of Mind-Body Health Sciences, Inc., in Scituate, Massachusetts.*

The message that underlies healing is simple yet radical: We are already whole. Underneath our fears and worries, unaffected by the many layers of our conditioning and actions, is a peaceful core. The work of healing is in peeling away the barriers of fear that keep us unaware of our true nature of love, peace, and rich interconnection with the web of life. Healing is the rediscovery of who we are and who we have always been.

It was written in Ecclesiastes that there is nothing new under the sun. As a medical scientist and psychologist interested in the interplay of unity that we see projected as the trinity of mind, body, and spirit, I would like to trace some of the current concepts in healing as they appeared in ancient texts and as they reappear in contemporary psychology and mind/body approaches to medicine.

Patanjali's *Yoga Sutras* are a compilation of philosophy, psychol-

ogy, and practical techniques of meditation and spiritual disciplines
that support healing. The central theme of healing is implicit in the
word *yoga,* which means "union." I like to think of this as a *reunion*
between the apparently time-limited self with whom we usually identify, and the limitless expression of a greater consciousness that most
of us experience in small glimpses—perhaps in the eyes of a child, in
the fragrance of a flower, or in the tears of remembrance that sometimes well up in response to music, art, or other expressions of the
sacred.

Compiled somewhere between 400 B.C. and A.D. 400, the sutras
—or "threads"—were core ideas that were memorized and handed
down through the millennia. Their basic ideas are common to many
philosophical systems and are found in the Upanishads centuries earlier. As we shall see, many of the same ideas have been rediscovered
in modern psychology.

If we define healing as an act of remembrance of who we already
are, we need to look at the attitudes that prevent us from realizing our
true nature, called the Atman or Self in the *Yoga Sutras.* These attitudes are referred to collectively as ignorance, and the perpetuation
of ignorance is defined as sin. In the yogic sense, sin is any thought
or act that keeps a person from recognizing his or her own inner
nature and its essential worthiness and connectedness to the larger
consciousness, or Godhead.

The essential aspect of yoga, according to Patanjali, is put forth
in the second sutra: "Yoga is the control of thought-waves in the
mind." Simply put, we are what we think. It is common to be sitting
in a comfortable room, surrounded by family, and yet be projecting
gloom and doom, which psychologists now call "awfulizing" or
"catastrophizing." Hordes of "if onlys" and "what ifs" close off the
possibility of enjoying the moment as it is.

Most of us are rarely in the present moment. Instead, we reside
in a thicket of past regrets and future fears, often based on the expectations of others. Nothing is ever good enough—especially us. Because
"now" is literally "the only time over which we have dominion," as
Tolstoy said, we are chronically selling out our own happiness and
contentment.

Yoga is an interconnected series of physical, emotional, mental,
and spiritual practices that lead to controlling the tyranny of the mind
and recognizing that the mind is an instrument that we use. It is *not*
who we are.

Every time the mind is still and we experience being in the

moment, we reconnect with the Self, the consciousness that enlivens the mind in the same way that electricity enlivens a light bulb. It is said that the mind is a wonderful servant but a terrible master. Modern cognitive psychology subscribes to similar tenets. We can learn to use our minds rather than to be used by them. To do this means learning to practice contentment.

STRESS AND PSYCHOLOGY

Stress is the password of the decade. It came under serious scrutiny by the medical establishment because of studies indicating that anywhere between 60 and 90 percent of the reasons people visit the family doctor are for "stress-related disorders" or problems such as colds or flu that will get better by themselves. Briefly stated, stress is the expectancy that bad things are going to happen and that we may not be able to cope with the fallout.

Thoughts of disaster immediately cause dramatic changes in the body's hormones and in the activity of its "overdrive system," called the sympathetic nervous system. A thought like, "Oh, God, I think that sound is a burglar!" activates a primitive circuit known as fight-or-flight. Heart rate and blood pressure skyrocket, sugar pours into the blood, muscles tense for quick action, and the whole metabolism rallies into a survival mode. This is great when we need it—but often we don't. When you activate the fight-or-flight circuit sitting in a traffic jam, thinking about your boss, composing nasty rejoinders to your spouse, or otherwise being in the grips of your mind, you begin to put needless wear and tear on the body. Research indicates that many modern maladies, from high blood pressure and headaches to digestive disorders and back pain, can be caused or worsened by stress.

Suzanne Kobasa, head of graduate psychology studies at the City University of New York, studies "stress-hardy" people. She and her colleague, Salvatore Maddi, studied a group of 2000 employees at a company that was undergoing divestiture. Some showed signs of stress—anxiety, depression, sleeplessness, poor health habits (people don't care much about the effects of smoking, drinking, and overeating when they feel "under the gun"), as well as stress-related physical problems such as headaches and ulcers. Other employees, however, coped beautifully and felt fine, regardless of the turmoil around them. Kobasa and Maddi studied these stress survivors and found that they had three important attitudes, the three Cs of stress-hardiness: challenge, commitment, and control.

Challenge refers to a frame of reference. Any event that disrupts the status quo can be seen either as a threat to things as they are or as a challenge to invent a new future. When we cling tightly to things as they are, any change looks like a threat. When we are open to the flow of possibilities, change looks like a challenge.

This is not a new understanding. There is an old Zen Buddhist aphorism, "Challenge is the correct way to view an inconvenience, and inconvenience is the incorrect way to view a challenge." There is, indeed, little new under the sun.

Commitment has to do with meaning. If we believe in what we are doing, the challenges we meet along the way are worthwhile; if we don't, the price is too great. People committed to their jobs, who believe in what they are doing, fare better than people who don't.

Viktor Frankl, in *Man's Search for Meaning*, tells how he endured the hideous atrocities of several Nazi death camps. He soon recognized that some people died quickly and others were survivors. Frequently, the survivors were those who found meaning in their experience. Frankl himself transformed the meaning of his suffering into the opportunity to be spokesperson for the importance of finding meaning in our lives.

Control is the biggest paradox of all. Psychologists have done elegant experiments showing that in rats a lack of control leads to ulcers and the inability to reject cancer, and in humans to anxiety, depression, and defects in the immune system. But what is control?

When we try to control everything in our lives, we lose sight of challenge because everything looks like a threat. Overcontrol leads to frustration, anger, and guilt. The Roman philosopher Epictetus reminded us that we would be forever miserable if we failed to distinguish between what was controllable and what wasn't. The Serenity Prayer used in the Anonymous programs offers similar wisdom: "God, grant me the serenity to accept the things I cannot change, the courage to change the things I can, and the wisdom to know the difference. Thy will, not mine, be done."

Kobasa's stress-hardiness research and theories of control are reminiscent of the ancient Kashmir Shaivite theories of human suffering. This ancient philosophy, also a yoga psychology, describes three great chains of bondage that cause us to suffer: imperfection, isolation, and control.

Imperfection is what psychologists discuss today under the rubric of self-esteem. In running a stress disorders program for the past six years, I can testify to the prevalence of thoughts about imperfection.

We are rarely "good enough." People who can marshal extraordinary compassion for others are often merciless with themselves. Think about this for a moment: When something goes wrong in your life, what do you say to yourself? Do you call yourself names? Maybe you call someone else names.

Blame is a sure-fire prescription for suffering. Psychologist Martin Seligman has defined the thought habits of pessimists (who, by the way, are much more likely to feel helpless and out of control than optimists). When something goes wrong in their lives, pessimists resort to reasons that are internal (they blame themselves), global (they think of how they fail generally, rather than thinking about the specific incident), and stable (they think the problem is typical of their lives, rather than seeing it as discrete in time). A pessimist who loses his job thinks that it is all his fault, it's the story of his whole life, and his flaws will last forever.

Isolation, the second chain of bondage in Kashmir Shaivism, refers to how we see ourselves as separate from the universe and from other people. This attitude is reflected in the tiresome inner dialogue over whether we are as good as, better than, or worse than others. Unfortunately, these kinds of thoughts intensify isolation.

Modern-day psychologists and sociologists see isolation as a health risk, as well as a cause of suffering. A large study in Alameda County, California, sought to determine the causes of poor health. Surprisingly, it was not socioeconomic status, how often people saw a doctor, or even smoking, drinking, exercise, and nutritional habits that were found to be the most important determinants of health. Instead, the study concluded that the more people who love us as part of our social network, the more healthy we are. Studies by Drs. Janice Kiecolt-Glaser and Ronald Glaser have shown that lonely people have more deficiencies in their immune systems compared to those who are not isolated.

Control, the third chain of bondage, is territory we've visited before. In the spiritual sense, control refers to the feeling that we are the center of the universe—the fear that the sun might not rise without our intervention. This is called being "the doer." It implies a lack of faith in the universe, and a resulting need to strangle everything to death by overcontrol. Guilty people, who suffer from a great deal of fear, fall squarely into this category. The doormats of the world, the long-suffering codependents of substance abusers, and many "do-gooders" who need to do good to cover up feelings of inadequacy, reap the fruits of this kind of suffering.

PEACE OF MIND

There are two great desires: to get what we want and to avoid what we don't want. As we all know, the best thing about a desire is when it stops—when we get what we want or get rid of what we don't want. For a moment, there is peace. That usually doesn't last long, however. Fueled by how good it felt to have a need met, the mind forms an association between contentment and the cessation of desires. We have to desire something else in order to feel satisfied. And so it goes, from one thing to the next. In the moment that the mind is still, residing in contentment, the "thought-waves" of Patanjali cease. When the mind becomes quiet, the underlying bliss of the Self is reexperienced. This great wheel of conditioning is how the whole case of mistaken identity gets its start.

The age-old prescription for retraining the mind is meditation, a kind of mental martial art in which, little by little, we realize that we are not our minds. In those few moments when the mind becomes calm, we experience a peacefulness, a contentment that is the inner Self, the part of our consciousness that is not conditioned by past experience. Because the body can be affected negatively by stress, it is not surprising that restoration of inner balance should be accompanied by a salubrious physiology that can reverse many stress-related illnesses.

Besides health benefits, meditation can give us a new way of dealing with our minds. Patanjali spoke of stilling the afflicting thought-waves in the mind by raising opposing thought-waves. This is called "thought stopping" in cognitive psychology. We become aware of the way the mind is torturing us, we decide to stop, and we substitute a better thought. Many of us use affirmations (I like to think of them as "station breaks" for the opposing point of view) that gradually dampen out the conditioned mind habits associated with suffering. As Patanjali says, however, eventually even the positive thoughts must be overcome, allowing us to enter more directly into the experience of being and the peace that is its hallmark.

THE DANGER OF SELF-BLAME

In our culture, many people have turned to meditation for its physiological benefits and have profited enormously. Nonetheless, we are all going to exit this planet through the mysterious portal called death. It is a fact of life that people forget all the time.

There currently seems to be a notion that if we eat right, exercise, meditate, and use visualization well enough, we will live forever. Obviously, our health habits do make a difference, but it is well to remember that even the great saints left their bodies—often from heart disease and cancer. I don't recall a single one lamenting that it would never have happened if they'd meditated better, imaged more vigorously, or forgone that last ice cream cone. Yet the tendency to blame ourselves is always rearing its ugly head.

Philosopher and author Ken Wilber calls this kind of thinking New Age narcissism. It is a resurrection of guilt and blame, one more expectation to which we think we have to conform. To think of illness as a form of punishment and healing as a reflection of our goodness traps us further in the Buddhist definition of suffering: the attachment to pleasure and the aversion to pain.

If we further believe that the state of our bodies reflects our self-worth, we are really doomed to suffering. Let us try to remember that the only definition of sin that makes any sense is this: any thought or deed that perpetuates our ignorance of our own intrinsic goodness. We are healed when we can grow from our suffering, when we can reframe it as an act of grace that leads us back to who we truly are.

Stephen Levine

THE HEALING FOR WHICH WE TOOK BIRTH

Stephen Levine, a poet, teacher of meditation, and former editor of the
San Francisco Oracle, *is coauthor (with Ram Dass) of* Grist for the
Mill *and has been a director of the Hanuman Foundation Dying Project.
He is widely known for his work with those confronting death and grief.
His book* Who Dies? *is often used by hospices and universities as a
teaching text.*

O ne way to approach the essential elements in healing is from the
standpoint of the suffering we all share, the place we feel unhealed. What we regard as suffering or as unhealed is partially a
question of perception, because much of what we call unhealed is that
to which we have resistance, such as pain.

Suppose you stub your toe. What kinds of energy have you been
conditioned to send into that throbbing discomfort? Most of us are
taught to send fear and anger, even hatred, into our pain. Which,
then, is the unhealed—the throbbing toe or the hateful response to
the unpleasant sensation?

Clearly, both factors are involved in our suffering. So true healing, which addresses the whole problem rather than partial manifesta-
tions, always involves meeting suffering with loving-kindness,
awareness, mercy, and balance, instead of trying to drive it away with
fear, distrust, anger, and loathing.

If we look into the mind and heart, we see that no remedy is more radical or more natural than to meet hatred and fear with mercy and loving-kindness. Even in the cases of people who have used powerful medicines to meet powerful illnesses—for example, chemotherapy or radiation treatment for cancer—we have seen that the real healing seems to have been marked by the ability to relinquish the suffering, to let the healing in. Indeed, in our work with dying patients, we have observed many examples of those who hated their treatment so much, who encapsulated their illness in such thick walls of resistance and fear, that it seemed a miracle if any of the chemotherapy or radiation could reach its target.

Healing, then, can be regarded as the establishment of a balance and equanimity in the midst of discomfort and agitation. We are healed when we can bring forth harmony out of the discordant strains of our life. And in my experience, one of the most effective ways of establishing such a balance and harmony is through care.

It is interesting to note that the word *care* is derived from the same root as *culture.* To bring oneself back into the common flow, the shared culture where the mind can relate to the body with heartfulness and mercy, is one of the bases of healing.

Another way of putting it is to say that an essential factor in all healing is love. For if the healer does not relate to that which calls out for healing with care, attention, and mercy—all aspects of love—then little healing can come about. Or, if there is "healing," it may be quite shallow, leaving the roots of the illness intact. Then the person "healed," although relieved of physical pain, remains with mental and spiritual pain untouched.

So many surface "healings" of this sort have left us unhealed. So many questions have been answered too quickly, thereby stopping the deeper investigation of the source of suffering in our lives. Often, it is discomfort in the body that puts us in touch with discomfort in the mind. To heal the body without including the mind, without allowing the body/mind to sink into the heart, is to continue the grief of a lifetime.

Another common denominator in the healing process is what I would call grace. But grace is a word much misunderstood. It is not a power that comes from without, from above, from elsewhere. Grace is our true nature; it is the source of healing that we carry within us.

So the closer we come to our true nature, the closer we come to the healing for which we took birth. Many, indeed most, people never focus on that profound inner healing power that seeks to bring balance to the mind so that the heart can shine through beyond hindrance or obstruction. In fact, for many people it is not until they experience a physical illness that they become concerned with the great inner healing faculty.

Real healing never stops. It cannot, for it is our birthright, our essential nature. It is the continuing expansion of the "big bang" of birth, constantly creating universes to be explored and merged into. To discover this inner grace in each moment is to become healed. It is to discover the human divine within, the very source of healing, the essence of the deathless, the ever-healed.

Some years ago, I worked with a woman who was hospitalized with bone metastasis, cancer that had infiltrated the bone and resulted, in her words, in a "burning agony." Her lifestyle and her way of relating to the world were such that she had mercilessly judged all those with whom she had come in contact. She had been a tough businesswoman and a difficult parent—to such a degree that, although she was apparently dying of cancer, her children would not visit her, having been pushed out of her heart and out of her life so often.

This woman had never met her grandchildren. Each nurse, doctor, or visitor who came into her room was greeted with anger and profanity. So she was usually alone in her misery, wrapped in self-pity and blaming others for her torment.

One night after six weeks in the hospital, when her pain was enormous, when the walls of resistance she had built to keep life and death away had become so strained that they could not withstand a moment's more pressure, the dam burst and her pain broke through. Then, perhaps for the first moment in her life, she drew a breath into her pain—a single breath. She surrendered for a moment and allowed the suffering to move through her, not resisting it as though it came from outside or was another's fault, but giving herself to it as her own.

She said later that in that moment—when the turbulent waters of her lifelong resistance and suffering broke through and swept over her as she lay on her side with enormous pain in her back, hips, and legs—she experienced herself not as that woman in the hospital, but as an Eskimo woman dying in childbirth. A moment later, she said, she was a black-skinned Biafran woman nursing a starving child from a slack breast, dying of hunger and disease. The next moment, she was another woman, lying beside a river in that same fetal position, her back crushed by a rockfall, dying alone.

Image after image arose, which she described afterwards as feeling the suffering of "ten thousand people in pain." After that experience, which broke her heart and brought her back into contact with herself, she realized, "It wasn't *my* pain; it was *the* pain. When it moved from 'my' pain to 'the' pain, it moved from the insufferable to the compassionate."

She had gone from the separate to the universal and had discovered that, when it is "my" pain, in this tiny mind and body, there is too little room for all that suffering. But when it is "the" pain, there is all the room in the world. Then the belly can remain soft, the heart can remain open, and our capacity to heal ourselves becomes the capacity to touch all the suffering in the world with mercy, loving-kindness, and a deeper sense of unity.

In the next six weeks, until she died, her room became the center of healing within the hospital. Many of the nurses spent their breaks there because it was the place where love was most radiant and evident. Within a week, after she had asked her children for forgiveness and pleaded for their return to her life, the grandchildren she had never met before were sitting next to her on the bed, playing "with Grandma . . . with Grandma's sweet, soft hands."

During those six weeks, the pain in her body diminished and the pain in her mind began to dissolve as her heart opened to encompass more and more life, more and more of that which is alive, and to touch the pain of all sentient beings with mercy and loving-kindness. We witnessed in that room one of the most remarkable healings we had ever seen. Although her body continued to deteriorate and she continued to be drawn gradually toward death, she died as healed as anyone we have ever seen.

Such healings have led us to investigate beyond the usual idea of healing—the idea of merely changing a dysfunction of the body—until now we see that healing goes far beyond the body to the very essence of that which inhabits the body: life itself, pure awareness, pure love.

We began this investigation with the realization that we didn't have the foggiest idea what healing really meant. Cases like the one described above led us to see that healing never stopped, and that the conventional ideas of healing were circumscribed by models in which healing was defined in terms of the body alone. But the body is in many ways "solidified mind." When the mind softens and mercy and compassion flood into the hard, cold areas of our being, which we have previously abandoned and feared, real healing begins.

Sometimes this process is reflected in a lessening of cancer or degenerative heart disease in the body. But often we see people "heal into death" in such a way that those around the deathbed are left with a sense of greater completion and wholeness; and we know the real healing will continue even after death.

One woman described her cancer as "the gift for the person who has everything." By this she meant that all her life she had looked for a teacher, a way through the mental and emotional pain that so often accompanied her desires and resistances to life. But it was not until she got cancer that she started to focus on the greater work to be done, on the healing for which she took birth.

Why do so many of us not give ourselves permission to be alive until we are absolutely assured that we will die? The healing we need is the healing that is all about us, to be found in this very instant, in this present millisecond of life and conscious experience. If we are not in that millisecond, we are not alive; we are merely thinking our lives. Yet we have seen so many die, looking back over their shoulders at their lives, shaking their heads and muttering in bewilderment, "What was that all about?"

John Lennon said, "Life is what's happening while we're busy making other plans." When healing becomes our priority, when being fully alive becomes a necessity instead of a mild, dilettantish interest, then real healing can occur. Most of the time, however, life seems not to be important or sufficient. Then we are always looking elsewhere for our satisfaction, forgetting that what we are looking for is that which is looking. And we forget that our healing comes in a willingness to be healed, a readiness to go beyond the old to something absolutely new and enter into the present moment with what Zen Master Sueng Sahn calls the great "Don't Know" Mind—a mind that has room for new possibilities and clings nowhere to the old.

All of this sounds good on paper, but it is often easier said than done. Simple though the technique is of bringing loving-kindness and a merciful awareness into that which has been rejected and shunned as ill or in need of healing, it is not always possible to accomplish it immediately. Yet what other choice do we have than to try to grow into our bodies?

Many of us who come to learn what "conscious dying" might be are really coming to discover how to be fully born. For, once we are fully born, death no longer is a problem but is seen more as a concept: not the opposite of life but as a moment within life, in the upward spiraling pattern of inner evolution that takes us to the very essence of healing and the healed.

In this journey of discovery, my wife, Ondrea, and I have been called on by the body to find the most practical kinds of application of these ideas and intuitions. Ondrea has twice been operated on for cancer. Indeed, when we met nine years ago, a medical person for whom we had great respect had told her she might well die within six months. As an acupuncturist, he had shown us how the stimulation of certain areas of the body might bring harmony and rebalance the energies necessary to rid her of both the side effects of surgery and the remaining cancerous cells. But because he lived a thousand miles away, it was not possible for us to visit him daily. He had, however, marked on her body the various points that should be treated.

So Ondrea and I began to practice acupuncture on her body daily. In my ineptitude and inexperience, I would often hit a nerve, causing a flash of fire to move through her body with a contraction and a slight cry of discomfort. I was causing pain to the person I most wanted not to be in pain! Sometimes we would both be crying as I turned a needle or inserted one deeper. Usually the wisdom of the body knew how and where to place the needles, but sometimes the difficulty we both experienced was considerable. Yet the love present in that room was so great and the desire for harmony so intense that something changed in her body.

Today, many years after that terminal prognosis, Ondrea's body is free of cancer, with no manifestation or symptoms in more than eight years. We still are not sure exactly what caused her body to change. The acupuncture helped, certainly, but we both feel that something more was involved. In fact, it is our sense that those needles acted almost like tiny antennae for the love in the room, for our care and concern for one another's well-being. Her body and my body were so closely merged in this conspiracy to meet in the heart of healing that healing was allowed in, through the needles, to the areas of pain and imbalance.

I would like to add, however, that I do not intend this example to short-circuit or limit the definition of healing. It is not meant to make readers feel, "If I was loved more, I might heal," or, "If I was handled with more care, I might be healed." Ondrea might well have died, for all we know, even if the conditions in the room had been no different. The very question "What is healing?" is not something that should be answered too quickly; it is only something in which one can participate with a sense of wonder and questioning that is never fully resolved. Like the truth, healing is not something to be known but something to be.

I have found this to be true in the healing of my own body as well. Born with congenital difficulties of the spine, I had several discs removed when I was nineteen years old. In the course of years, three more discs in my neck collapsed and for a while I was in considerable pain. Then, remembering the investigation that Ondrea and I had started with the cancer in her body, we put great amounts of time into focusing on sending mercy and loving-kindness into the problem in my body. Over a period of some months, the area—which various doctors said would only be cured by surgery—seemed to soften and open to healing. The numbness in both my arms eased, as well as inability to sleep because of pain. Now instead of pain I feel a quiet mercy that is sometimes a soreness but is usually an open spaciousness, reminiscent of the sense Ondrea and I both experienced in the chest when our hearts were open and it seemed as though heaven and earth were meeting within the body, mind, and heart.

One key to developing the sensitivity that allows one to open to healing in this way is the practice of meditation. In the role of healer or therapist, one can become so sensitive in deeper levels of meditation practice that one's body can become like a fine-tuned diagnostic instrument. Then by feeling various changes in one's body and mind while with a client, one can understand something deeper of the client's inner experience and illness. Many techniques and therapies are useful, but nothing is as effective as daily meditation practice to deepen the well from which the thirst for healing may be slaked. Meditation develops the sensitivity needed to use any method of healing with skill and effectiveness.

For this reason, the particular technique used by a healer is almost beside the point. Having worked with thousands of terminally ill people, I must say in all honesty that I do not see any technique that is outstandingly better than any other. So much depends on the individual's temperament and willingness to heal and be healed. We have an enormous bookshelf at home full of hundreds of books on different healing procedures and systems—flower remedies, acupuncture, standard surgery, radiation, chemotherapy, fever therapy, urine therapy, wheat-grass therapies, crystal therapies, light therapies, color therapies. Yet all of these books were used by various patients at times in their illnesses and were left to us after their deaths.

In each book I see a few shining examples of hearts that have opened beyond pain, people who have moved into their own healing and resolved conflict in the heart of perfect understanding and love. So it seems that it is not the techniques that set us free; it is not what we do, but how we do it.

Grasping at healing, like grasping at enlightenment, results in unbearable suffering, for all grasping results in distress. But to allow ourselves to lighten, to allow ourselves to heal, to trust the process and enter into it without models or preconceptions of how we're supposed to be or who we're supposed to be, seems to be the very path that Healing and Light travel. When we remember that we are the path and that we must tread it ourselves—lightly, mercifully, and consciously—then the healing that goes beyond "healing" becomes our birthright, and we truly discover ourselves.

AFTERWORD

T he attempt to help uncover the golden thread of healing does not
end with the completion of this book. What we had hoped to
accomplish was to weave an unfinished tapestry. The strands laid
down by the contributing authors have endured through the ages. It
is up to each of you to continue to weave threads into a larger work
that creates your personal vision.

Every field of knowledge seems to be aided by an understanding
of the essential elements involved. The field of healing is no exception. As more healing techniques are developed each year, it will
become increasingly important to come back to the fundamental basis
of healing. In other words, by not getting lost in individual techniques, we can discover, or perhaps rediscover, what healing is really
about.

Perhaps the greatest gift our authors have given us is an enhanced sense that we are all healers. Effective healing does not necessarily stem from an increased education or mastery of technique.
Rather, healing can take place when one or more persons open their
hearts and spirits to the gifts they already possess.

BENJAMIN SHIELD
RICHARD CARLSON
P.O. Box 1196
Orinda, CA 94563

About the Editors

Benjamin Shield is a Rolfer and cranio-sacral therapist practicing in Santa Monica, California. He holds B.S. degrees in biochemistry and biology from the University of California at Santa Barbara and has done postgraduate work at Boston University School of Medicine. His primary focus is directed toward going beyond technique, searching for the common denominators or "golden threads" of healing.

Richard Carlson, Ph.D., holds a doctoral degree in psychology from Sierra University, San Francisco, California. He is an author and advocate in the areas of self-improvement and spiritual growth. He maintains a private practice in Oakland, California, where he lives with his wife, Kristine. His primary goal is to teach the role that attitude can play in a person's healing process.